Manual for the
SEMISTRUCTURED CLINICAL INTERVIEW FOR CHILDREN AND ADOLESCENTS

Stephanie H. McConaughy
Thomas M. Achenbach
Department of Psychiatry
University of Vermont

Ordering Information

This book and all materials related to the Semistructured Clinical Interview for Children and Adolescents can be ordered from:

University Associates in Psychiatry
1 South Prospect St.
Burlington, VT 05401-3456
Fax: 802/656-2602

Proper bibliographic citation for this book:

McConaughy, S.H., & Achenbach, T.M. (1994). *Manual for the Semistructured Clinical Interview for Children and Adolescents.* Burlington, VT: University of Vermont Department of Psychiatry.

Related Books

Achenbach, T.M. (1991). *Integrative guide for the 1991 CBCL/4-18, YSR, and TRF profiles.* Burlington, VT: University of Vermont Department of Psychiatry.

Achenbach, T.M. (1991). *Manual for the Child Behavior Checklist/4-18 and 1991 Profile.* Burlington, VT: University of Vermont Department of Psychiatry.

Achenbach, T.M. (1991). *Manual for the Teacher's Report Form and 1991 Profile.* Burlington, VT: University of Vermont Department of Psychiatry.

Achenbach, T.M. (1991). *Manual for the Youth Self-Report and 1991 Profile.* Burlington, VT: University of Vermont Department of Psychiatry.

Achenbach, T.M. (1992). *Manual for the Child Behavior Checklist/2-3 and 1992 Profile.* Burlington, VT: University of Vermont Department of Psychiatry.

Achenbach, T.M. (1993). *Empirically based taxonomy: How to use syndromes and profile types derived from the CBCL/4-18, TRF, and YSR.* Burlington, VT: University of Vermont Department of Psychiatry.

Library of Congress #94-60044 ISBN 0-938565-32-X

Printed in the United States of America 12 11 10 9 8 7 6 5 4 3 2 1

USER QUALIFICATIONS

The *Semistructured Clinical Interview for Children and Adolescents* (SCICA) is designed for ages 6 to 18. Eligibility to use the SCICA requires specific training in clinical interviewing of children and adolescents, as well as knowledge of the theory and methodology of standardized assessment. Our standards for use are consistent with the *Standards for Educational and Psychological Testing* (AERA et al., 1985) endorsed by the American Educational Research Association (AERA), American Psychological Association (APA), and National Council on Measurement in Education (NCME). Users are expected to adhere to the ethical principles of the American Psychological Association or National Association of School Psychologists.

We require all purchasers of the SCICA to furnish evidence of their qualifications by completing a User Registration available from the authors. Administration of the SCICA requires *(1)* graduate training in standardized assessment commensurate with at least the Master's degree in psychology, social work, or special education, or two years of residency in pediatrics or psychiatry; and *(2)* supervised experience in interviewing children and adolescents. The user must have sufficient prior experience with diverse children of the ages to be interviewed to be comfortable talking with them and to handle the many unexpected events that may occur. Trainees under the supervision of a qualified professional may qualify for purchasing the SCICA if both supervisor and supervisee sign the User Registration.

USER QUALIFICATIONS

A qualified individual user or supervisor must be identified for all institutional purchases of SCICA materials.

The SCICA should not be the sole basis for making diagnoses or other important decisions about children and adolescents. No item or score on the SCICA should be automatically equated with any particular diagnosis or inferred disorder. Instead, the SCICA is intended to be used in conjunction with standardized procedures for obtaining information from other sources. The responsible professional will compare the data obtained from the SCICA with data from other sources, such as parents, teachers, standardized tests, medical and developmental history, and direct observations in other settings. To administer and interpret the SCICA properly, the user should have thorough knowledge of the procedures and cautions presented in this *Manual*.

PREFACE

This *Manual* provides basic information needed for understanding and using the SCICA. The *Manual* includes information on the background, rationale, development, and use of the SCICA, current research on reliability and validity, applications of the SCICA, case illustrations, and examples of formats for integrating SCICA results with other assessment information. To date, we have developed empirically based scales for the SCICA scoring profile for ages 6-12. The SCICA Protocol Form contains questions and tasks applicable to ages from 6 to 18, plus specific questions for adolescents. Research is under way to develop a SCICA scoring profile for ages 13-18.

In developing the SCICA over the last decade, we have benefitted from the help and advice of many colleagues as well as the subjects, their families, and school staff who have cooperated in our research. In particular, we are grateful for the assistance of Neil Aguiar, Janet Arnold, Judy Ewell, Elizabeth Flannery, Cathleen Gent, David Jacobowitz, Marianne Kazius, Cynthia LaRiviere, Virginia MacDonald, Barry Nurcombe, Amy Ojerholm, Vicky Phares, David Rettew, Catherine Stanger, Kelly Ahn Starr, James Tallmadge, and Andrew Weine. We have appreciated the advice of our colleagues James Hudziak, Hans Koot, David Van Buskirk, and Frank Verhulst regarding our interviewing and training procedures. The work reported here has been supported by University Associates in Psychiatry, a nonprofit health services and research corporation of the University of Vermont Department of Psychiatry. We are also grateful to the Spencer Foundation, W. T. Grant Foundation, and National Institute on Disability and Rehabilitation Research (U.S. Department of Education) for support of research that has contributed to this effort.

READER'S GUIDE

CONTENTS

Chapter 1
Rationale for the Semistructured Clinical Interview for Children and Adolescents

This *Manual* is a revised and extended version of our *Guide to the Semistructured Clinical Interview for Children* (McConaughy & Achenbach, 1990). Our interview is now called the *Semistructured Clinical Interview for Children and Adolescents* (SCICA) to reflect the extension of our procedures to age 18. The SCICA Protocol Form and SCICA Observation and Self-Report Forms include questions and items to be scored for subjects aged 6 to 18. The 1994 SCICA Profile covers ages 6-12, but we plan to provide a version for ages 13-18 after further research. This *Manual* reports results of our research to develop the SCICA protocol, rating forms, and scoring profile for ages 6-12.

Small changes have been made in the wording of some items from the 1990 Observation and Self-Report Forms. Certain items have also been moved and renumbered in order to include new items derived from our research and to add items appropriate for ages 13-18. With the new SCICA computer program, users can obtain scores on the 1994 SCICA Profile from data previously entered via the 1990 SCIC computer program.

ORGANIZATION OF THIS MANUAL

To aid readers who are unfamiliar with the SCICA, as well as readers who are familiar with the 1990 version, this *Manual* describes our rationale for developing the SCICA within the context of a multiaxial assessment model.

1

Chapter 1 reviews previous research on structured and semistructured interviews and contrasts this with the psychometric approach we used to develop the SCICA. The SCICA protocol, rating forms, and scoring profile are described in Chapter 2. Chapter 3 offers guidelines for interviewing children and describes training procedures we have developed. Chapter 4 presents the research basis for the SCICA rating forms and profile, including statistical derivation of the SCICA scales and assignment of standard scores. Chapters 5 and 6 present reliability and validity data. Chapter 7 presents relations between the 1994 SCICA and the previous 1990 SCIC scales, while Chapter 8 presents relations between the SCICA and other empirically based assessment procedures. Applications of the SCICA to various assessment tasks are outlined in Chapter 9. Chapter 10 presents case illustrations and a sample report that combines results from the SCICA with other data. Chapter 11 provides answers to commonly asked questions about the SCICA and its role in multiaxial empirically based assessment.

Instructions for scoring the SCICA Observation and Self-Report items are provided in Appendix A. Appendix B lists the items and their loadings from principal components analyses for the eight empirically derived syndromes of the 1994 SCICA Profile for Ages 6-12. Appendix C presents means and standard deviations of SCICA scale scores for matched referred and nonreferred samples. Correlations among SCICA scale scores are presented in Appendix D.

ADVANTAGES OF INTERVIEWS
WITH CHILDREN

Clinical interviews are widely used as a basis for diagnosing disorders and formulating treatment plans for children. Interviews are often used by psychiatrists, clinical psychologists, school psychologists, social workers, and other mental health workers. Even experts in behavioral assessment stress the importance of interviews as key components of multimethod approaches to evaluating children's problems (Hughes & Baker, 1990).

Clinicians feel that interviews are essential for obtaining first-hand impressions of children's affective and interpersonal functioning. For example, Hughes (1989) described the following advantages of child interviews for clinical assessments: *(1)* they provide opportunities for assessing children's coping strategies and perceptions of significant persons and events related to their problems; *(2)* they enable the interviewer to observe behavior that may be relevant to the choice of treatment options; *(3)* they can tap areas of functioning that may be less amenable to other assessment procedures; and *(4)* they can help to establish the rapport necessary for effective treatment.

Despite the importance of child interviews, poor agreement on diagnoses by different interviewers has led to accusations that child clinical interviews are "quasi-scientific" and that they produce biased results (see Young, O'Brien, Gutterman, & Cohen, 1987). To counter such charges, structured and semistructured interviews were developed to standardize procedures (for reviews, see Gutterman, O'Brien, & Young, 1987; Hodges, 1993). By more precisely defining question and response formats, researchers hoped to reduce information variance and thereby improve the reliability and validity of child interviews. Structured parent interviews were also developed to provide an additional source of data on children's problems. Such interviews have been thought to have the following advantages: *(1)* they provide opportunities to obtain child interview data in a systematic manner; *(2)* they ensure that broad ranges of symptoms and diagnoses are assessed; and *(3)* parallel child and parent interviews provide systematic comparisons of child and parent reports for the same symptoms (Hughes & Baker, 1990; Witt, Cavell, Carey, & Martens, 1988).

Structured and semistructured interviews have become major data sources for epidemiologic research on the prevalence of childhood psychiatric disorders. In reviewing such research, Hodges (1993) drew the following conclusions: *(1)* many children and adolescents can respond meaningfully to direct questions about their mental status; *(2)* there is no evidence that asking children such questions increases their risk for psychopathology; *(3)* low to moderate agreement between children and parents indicates that these two informants are not interchangeable; *(4)* structured interviews can be used to assess comorbidity between different psychiatric diagnoses; *(5)* structured interviews must be supplemented by measures of general functioning or impairment to determine need for treatment; and *(6)* extensive training is required to obtain acceptable reliability, even when interviewers are experienced clinicians. To familiarize readers with prior research on child interviews, the major features of structured and semistructured interviews are reviewed in the following sections.

STRUCTURED INTERVIEWS

Several structured diagnostic interviews have been developed since the 1960s. The interviews vary from highly structured to less structured formats. Highly structured interviews require strict adherence to standardized procedures for asking questions, recording responses, and sequencing of items. Examples are the *Diagnostic Interview for Children and Adolescents* (DICA; Herjanic & Reich, 1982; DICA-R; Reich & Welner, 1992) and the *NIMH Diagnostic Interview Schedule for Children* (DISC; Costello, Edelbrock, Dulcan, Kalas, & Klaric, 1984; DISC-2.3; Shaffer, 1992). Less structured interviews also use standard question formats, but allow the interviewer to adjust the length and sequence of items to fit the characteristics of the child and to create a more conversational approach. Examples are the *Interview Schedule for Children* (ISC; Kovacs, 1983) and

Schedule for Affective Disorders and Schizophrenia for School-Aged Children (Kiddie-SADS or K-SADS; Ambrosini, Metz, Prabucki, & Lee, 1989; Puig-Antich & Chambers, 1978). The current versions of all four interviews provide separate forms for interviewing the child and parent. The DICA-R has separate versions for young children and adolescents.

The DICA, DISC, ISC, and K-SADS share several features. First, they employ standard sets of questions and response categories, usually involving a branching hierarchy of questions and probes. That is, within different content categories, questions are arranged with skip procedures such that the choice of the next question depends on the respondent's answer to the question that preceded it. Questions and probes vary in number across interviews, ranging from 200 on the ISC to over 1,500 on the DISC 2.3.

A second feature shared by the four structured interviews is that they generate DSM diagnoses (*Diagnostic and Statistical Manual of Mental Disorders*; American Psychiatric Association, DSM-III, 1980; DSM-III-R, 1987; DSM-IV, 1994). Although diagnoses vary across interviews, most include common diagnoses attributed to children, such as attention deficit disorder, conduct disorders, oppositional defiant disorder, depression, dysthymia, and anxiety disorders. Some of the interviews also contain additional items for screening psychotic symptoms, substance abuse, and less common diagnoses.

A third feature of the structured interviews is dichotomous scoring of diagnoses as present versus absent according to whether criteria have been met. Individual items or symptoms may be scored as "present versus absent" or on 3- to 7-point scales (e.g., DISC-2.3 items are scored as "no," "sometimes/somewhat," "yes," or "don't know"). Scores for individual items or symptoms are then aggregated according to computer algorithms or clinical judgments to obtain a yes/no decision for each diagnosis.

The structured interviews differ in the length of time required for administration and in the experience required of the interviewer. All four interviews require at least 45 to 60 minutes for administration, but some can take as long as 4 to 6 hours, depending on the number of symptoms reported by the respondent. The ISC and K-SADS must be administered by experienced clinicians, whereas the DICA-R and DISC 2.3 were designed for lay interviewers. Regardless of whether interviewers are experienced clinicians or lay persons, extensive training is required to achieve acceptable levels of reliability (Costello, Burns, Angold, & Leaf, 1993; Hodges, 1993).

Another difference is that the DICA and the DISC can be considered "respondent-based" interviews in contrast to "interviewer-based" approaches, which characterize the ISC and K-SADS. In respondent-based interviews, the respondent's answers to structured questions comprise the data retained from the interview. In interviewer-based interviews, the interviewer's judgments about the respondent's answers to questions comprise the data. The DISC, for example, was modelled on the *Diagnostic Interview Schedule* (DIS; Robins, Helzer, Cottler, & Goldring, 1989) used in the adult Epidemiological Catchment Area (ECA) studies. As Costello et al. (1993) explain, the aim of the DIS and DISC was "to structure the behavior of the interviewers in such a way that the 'stimulus' presented to each respondent was as similar as possible" (p. 1110). The DIS and DISC were thus designed to reduce variability across interviews by standardizing the interaction between the interviewer and respondent. The respondent-based approach was intended to limit the range of responses to similar sets of questions for all respondents, whose answers to the questions comprise the essential data obtained from the interview. In this respect, according to Costello et al., the DIS and DISC are similar to long questionnaires administered verbally.

"Interviewer-based" approaches, by contrast, allow for more flexibility in questioning techniques. They also require clinical judgments for determining the presence of symptoms and diagnoses. The ISC and K-SADS can be considered interviewer-based approaches, owing to their reliance on experienced clinicians for more open-ended interviewing and formulation of diagnoses. Purer examples of interviewer-based approaches are found among the semistructured interviews discussed next.

SEMISTRUCTURED INTERVIEWS

Semistructured interviews are less rigid in their format than structured interviews. The semistructured interviews employ open-ended questions that can be followed by probes when appropriate. The interviewer can alter questions and vary the sequence of topics to follow the child's natural flow of conversation. Some semistructured interviews also include nonverbal activities, such as drawing and play materials, to provide more options for interacting and establishing rapport with the child. Examples of semi-structured interviews are the *Child Assessment Schedule* (CAS; Hodges, McKnew, Cytryn, Stern, & Kline, 1982; Hodges, Cools, & McKnew, 1989; Hodges, Gordon, & Lennon, 1990); the *Child and Adolescent Psychiatric Assessment* (CAPA; Angold, Cox, Prendergast, Rutter, & Simonoff, 1987; Angold & Costello, 1993); the *Isle of Wight Inventory* (IWI; Rutter & Graham, 1968); the *Mental Health Assessment Form* (MHAF; Kestenbaum & Bird, 1978); and the *Social Adjustment Inventory for Children and Adoles-cents* (SAICA; John, Gammon, Prusoff, & Warner, 1987).

Like the structured interviews, most semistructured interviews yield clinical diagnoses. The CAS and the CAPA, in particular, are designed to produce DSM diagnoses. The CAPA also produces ICD diagnoses (International Classification of Diseases; World Health Organization, 1992). In addition, the semistructured interviews yield scores for content areas, mental status, affect, observed behavior, and global ratings of psychopathology or total pathology scores. Scoring systems for semistructured interviews generally include present versus absent ratings and/or multi-step scales for rating the severity of problems.

The CAS (Hodges et al., 1989; Hodges et al., 1990) is intended to combine the standardized procedures of structured interviews with the flexibility of semistructured interviews. Separate versions are used for interviewing children and parents. The CAS consists of 320 items organized into three broad sections. First, the interviewer asks the child open-ended questions concerning school, friends, activities, hobbies, family, and groupings of psychiatric symptoms. Questions are organized according to 11 content areas so that the interviewer can vary the sequence of topics to match the child's conversation. After completing all of the content areas, the interviewer asks specific questions about the onset and duration of symptoms that were reported to be present. In a third section, after the interview is completed, the interviewer rates the child on 53 items covering behavior, affect, interpersonal interactions, and estimated cognitive ability, based on observations during the interview. Each CAS item is scored as "yes," "no," "ambiguous," or "unscorable." Response items are phrased such that a "yes" always indicates the presence of a symptom. The CAS can be scored by hand or computer to obtain a total pathology score, as well as scores for the content areas, symptom scales, and DSM diagnoses.

The CAPA (Angold et al., 1987) is a semistructured interview for children aged 8 to 18. There are separate versions for interviewing children and their parents. The general format is semistructured, consisting of open-ended questions that introduce a particular topic area, followed by more specific probes tapping details of each topic for later scoring by the interviewer. The interview is divided into three broad sections: introduction, symptom review, and incapacity ratings. The introduction, which is intended to establish rapport, includes general questions regarding home and family life, school, peer groups, and spare time activities. The symptom review involves detailed questions about specific symptoms or problems that comprise 17 domains corresponding to psychiatric diagnoses. The CAPA protocol lists a definition of each symptom or problem followed by open-ended questions and probes regarding each symptom.

The interviewer must cover all symptoms, but can address sets of symptoms organized in a modular fashion (e.g., anxiety disorders, oppositional and conduct disorders, school-related problems, etc.), starting with areas thought to be problematic for a particular child, as inferred from the child's responses in the introductory section. Following the symptom review, the interviewer questions the child about the effects of each reported symptom on 17 areas of "incapacity," such as relationships with parents, relationships with peers, homework, spare time activities, etc. The interviewer must establish whether an "incapacity" is secondary to particular symptoms reported earlier (e.g., the child's reported loss of friends is due to a fear of leaving the home), rather than to some other factor separate from the symptom (e.g., the child's reported loss of friends is due to a move to a new community).

After the CAPA is completed, the interviewer scores the CAPA items according to a glossary of definitions for each symptom and incapacity. The symptoms are scored for duration, frequency, time of onset, and intensity. Most CAPA items are rated on the basis of the 3 months preceding the interview, except for certain infrequent problems involving discrete acts, such as setting fires or suicidal behavior. Duration is coded as the length of time (in hours or minutes) of the average "bout" (episode of continuous occurrence) of a symptom during the preceding 3 months. Frequency is coded as the number of symptom bouts or discrete acts over the same period. Intensity is scored on 4-point scales according to criteria defined for each item. The interviewer judges whether the specific scoring criteria are met. In addition to the symptom and incapacity ratings, the interviewer scores 67 observational items for activity level, mood, quality of social interaction, and psychotic behavior.

Computer algorithms aggregate the interviewer's ratings to produce present or absent scores for some 40 DSM or ICD diagnoses, as well as providing scores for the number of symptoms reported for each diagnosis and incapacity scores for each diagnosis. An optional section of the CAPA assesses critical life events impinging on the child's problems, while a companion interview has also been developed for assessing service utilization (Burns, Angold, Macgruder-Habib, Costello, & Patrick, 1992).

The IWI (Rutter & Graham, 1968) and the MHAF (Kestenbaum & Bird, 1978) are semistructured interviewer-based interviews designed for children aged 7 to 12. Both interviews cover important life areas, such as relationships with family members, activities, and school, as well as specific questions concerning psychiatric symptoms or mental status. Question formats are suggested, but the exact wording of questions is left up to the interviewer to adapt to the child's cognitive level and interaction style. The interviewer records the child's responses during the interview and notes observed behavior and affect.

After the IWI or MHAF is completed, the interviewer scores the child on specific items describing psychiatric symptoms or aspects of mental status exhibited by the child during the interview. For the IWI, the interviewer rates the child on 21 items describing behavior and affect, using 3-point scales. The interviewer also makes a global judgment as to whether the child showed no, slight, or marked overall psychiatric abnormality. For the MHAF, the interviewer rates the child on 189 items describing aspects of mental status (appearance, behavior, relatedness, affect, language, etc.), as well as the content of the issues discussed during the interview. The interviewer scores each item according to whether the interviewer thinks the child deviates from the "norm" expected for the child's age, using 5-point and 7-point scales. A global score is also obtained from the MHAF for overall psychopathology. Both the IWI and MHAF produced high inter-rater reliabilities for judgments of overall psychopathology ($r \geq .80$), but reliabilities have varied considerably for specific psychiatric symptoms, aspects of behavior, and mental status (Kestenbaum & Bird, 1978; Rutter & Graham, 1968). Unlike the CAPA and CAS, the IWI and the MHAF were not designed to produce specific DSM or ICD diagnoses.

The SAICA (John et al., 1987) is called a semistructured interview, but it differs from other interviews in several respects. The SAICA includes both problem behaviors and competence items chosen to tap four role areas: school, spare time activities, peer relations, and home functioning. After each question, the interviewer asks the child to select which one of four possible ratings best describes the child's behavior. The interviewer may probe for more information, but the child's judgment, rather than the interviewer's, is scored. After completing the interview, the interviewer makes global ratings of the child's competence and problem behaviors in each of the four role areas. Factor analyses of the SAICA yielded three factors designated as School and Spare Time Activities, Spare Time Sociability, and Family Relations, which cut across the four *a priori* role areas. The total score on the SAICA successfully discriminated dysthymic children from children receiving no diagnosis, but did not discriminate any other diagnosis from no diagnosis.

LIMITATIONS OF CURRENT INTERVIEWS

Despite their value for clinical practice and research, the existing structured and semistructured interviews have several limitations. Major limitations include formats that are inappropriate for children and have led to poor test-retest reliabilities, heavy dependence on DSM (or ICD) diagnoses as the primary product of the interview, and a lack of procedures for integrating data from different sources. These limitations and related issues are discussed in the following sections.

Inappropriate Interview Formats for Children

A major limitation of many structured and semistructured interviews is their incompatibility with children's cognitive level and interaction styles. The length and detail of such interviews can pose formidable challenges to young children's attention span and tolerance for verbal questioning. Adolescents experiencing emotional or behavioral problems may also have trouble tolerating long, rigid interviews. Even the interviewers themselves may find it hard to carry out complicated questioning and recording of responses while observing and maintaining rapport with the interviewee.

Structured Interviews. Inappropriate formats are a particular problem for the respondent-based structured interviews. To standardize procedures across subjects, the respondent-based interviews use exactly the same questions with all children, regardless of age or cognitive level. As Costello et al. (1993) point out, this approach assumes that children, regardless of their developmental level, will "(1) understand the questions in the same way, (2) be equally capable of deciding whether they have experienced the phenomenon in question, and (3) be equally capable of deciding whether the level at which they experienced it falls into the range of deviance that interests the interviewer" (p. 1110).

The inappropriateness of structured interview formats has been reflected in findings of lower reliability and stability of symptom scores for younger children than for adolescents. For example, Edelbrock, Costello, Dulcan, Kalas, and

Conover (1985) obtained 9-day test-retest correlations of only .39 at ages 6 to 9 and .55 at ages 10 to 13, versus .81 at ages 14 to 18 for total symptom scores on the child version of the DISC. In contrast, 9-day test-retest correlations for total symptom scores from parent versions of the DISC were .90 for the 6-9-year-olds and .78 for the 10-13-year-olds. The child version of the DICA-R also produced much lower test-retest kappas (a measure of agreement for categorical data) for DSM diagnoses for 6-11-year-olds than for 12-16-year-olds (Boyle et al., 1993).

Along with lower test-retest reliabilities, Edelbrock et al. (1985) reported that young children seemed to employ a yea-saying set (i.e., responding "yes" to many symptoms) to initial DISC interviews and then switched to a nay-saying set (i.e., responding "no" to many of the same symptoms) in retest interviews. The researchers surmised that the change from yea-saying to nay-saying occurred because children had learned that negative responses shortened the interview process. This produced large declines in child-reported symptom scores from Time 1 to Time 2.

Because of the lower reliabilities obtained for young children, the DISC-2.3 is now recommended only for children aged 9-17 (Shaffer, 1992). Nonetheless, declines in DISC symptoms from Time 1 to Time 2 (*attenuation effects*) and lower test-retest reliabilities for younger than for older children have been found even for respondents above age 9. For example, test-retest kappas were significantly lower for 9-12-year-olds than for 13-18-year-olds for diagnoses of depression/dysthymia and conduct disorder, based on DISC-2 child interviews of community samples (Jensen, Roper, Fisher, & Piacenti, 1994). The tendency for subjects to report fewer symptoms at Time 2 than Time 1 did more to reduce test-retest reliability than did any other respondent characteristics, such as impulsive answers, being slow to warm up, or endorsement of many symptoms by "noncases" (Jensen et al., 1994). Such attenuation effects have not been limited to the DISC, since the CAPA also showed test-retest declines in symptom scores for all diagnoses, except major depression. Differences between Time 1 and Time 2 CAPA symptom scores were not significant, but this was probably due to small sample sizes for the different diagnostic areas (Ns ranging from 5 to 23).

Semistructured Interviews. The more flexible format of the semistructured interviews was intended to accommodate to children's interaction styles and thereby improve reliability. On the CAS, this approach yielded a 5-day test-retest correlation of .89 for total symptom scores among 6- to 12-year-old inpatients. Test-retest kappas for diagnoses were also better with the CAS (Hodges et al., 1989) than with an early version of the DISC (Costello et al., 1984). Compared to the later DISC-2 (Jensen et al., 1994), the CAS yielded better test-retest reliabilities for diagnoses of anxiety disorders and depression/dysthymia, but comparable reliabilities for conduct disorder and attention deficit disorder in clinic samples. It is possible, however, that the more severe psychopathology in the inpatient sample used to test the CAS contributed to the higher reliability found with the CAS than with the DISC, for which outpatient clinic samples and community samples were used to test reliability.

Differences among Diagnoses

Test-retest reliabilities for structured and semistructured interviews have varied according to diagnoses. In general, test-retest kappas have been relatively high (>.60) for diagnoses of conduct disorders derived from the most recent child versions of the CAS, DISC, and ISC (Jensen et al., 1994; Hodges, 1993), as well as adolescent versions of the DICA-R (Boyle et al., 1993). Kappas have also been relatively high (>.70) for diagnoses of depression/dysthymia on child versions of the CAS and ISC (Hodges, 1993), but low on the DISC-2 (kappas = .29 to .38; Jensen et al., 1994) and DICA-R (kappa = .21; Boyle et al., 1993). Kappas for diagnoses of anxiety disorders and attention deficit disorders have varied from low to high across interviews. Test-retest kappas for the child version of the CAPA ranged from .54 for conduct disorder to .90 for major depression and 1.0 for substance use/dependence (Angold & Costello, 1993). Intraclass correlations computed between Time 1 and Time 2 CAPA symptom scores for each diagnosis ranged from .50 for oppositional defiant disorder to .85 for major depression and .95 for substance use/dependence.

Dependence on DSM Diagnoses

Dependence on DSM diagnoses as the primary product is another limitation of many structured and semistructured interviews. The close tie to the DSM makes such interview formats vulnerable to the frequent revisions of the DSM. Interviewers also require extensive training in differential diagnosis according to the current version of the DSM (Costello et al., 1993; Young et al., 1987). Furthermore, categorical DSM diagnoses tell us little about children's thoughts or feelings about their problems, their understanding of the causes of problems, problems that are omitted from the DSM criteria, or the contexts where problems occur, all of which are important for assessment and treatment.

A related limitation is that most structured and semistructured interviews rely on present versus absent scores for symptoms and diagnoses. Although symptoms may be scored initially on more differentiated scales, the diagnostic algorithms require categorization of each symptom as present or absent and each child as a "case" or "noncase" for each diagnosis, based on fixed cutpoints for diagnostic criteria. The sensitivity (percent of correctly identified cases) and specificity (percent of correctly identified noncases) depends on the cutpoint used to identify cases (Rey, Morris-Yates, & Stanislaw, 1992; Young et al, 1987). Dichotomous categorization according to cutpoints can lose important information regarding the severity of problems.

For example, children who just met the minimum diagnostic criteria required for making a DSM-III diagnosis from the parent version of the DISC obtained significantly lower problem scores on the Child Behavior Checklist (CBCL) than did children who exceeded the minimum criteria required for a diagnosis (Edelbrock & Costello, 1988). This indicated that there were important quantitative differences in problems among children who all met criteria for a particular DSM diagnosis.

Categorization according to DSM diagnoses can also mask the variety of problems found in many children. This occurs because a particular diagnosis provides information only about the symptoms associated with that diagnosis. It does not include information about other problems that may exist but are not associated with that diagnosis and do not qualify for an additional diagnosis. For example, Edelbrock and Costello (1988) found that DSM diagnoses of depression and dysthymia, based on DISC parent interviews, correlated significantly with both Internalizing and Externalizing scores on the CBCL. The categorical diagnoses of depression and dysthymia, however, did not reflect the Externalizing problems also exhibited by the children.

Lack of Procedures for Integrating Multi-Source Data

Categorical diagnoses generated from a single source, such as a child interview, are often difficult to integrate with the discrepant data obtained from other sources. Diagnoses based on separate interviews of children and their parents have generally shown only low to moderate agreement (for reviews, see Hodges, 1993; Young et al., 1987). Parent-child agreement has typically been moderate to high for externalizing symptoms, moderate for depressive symptoms, and low for anxiety symptoms (Edelbrock, Costello, Dulcan, Conover, & Kalas, 1986; Hodges, 1993; Hodges, Gordon, & Lennon, 1990). Such findings have raised questions about the validity of child diagnoses obtained from interviews.

However, low to moderate parent-child agreement is consistent with the modest cross-informant agreement found in ratings of behavioral and emotional problems (Achenbach, McConaughy, & Howell, 1987). Low parent-child agreement does not necessarily mean that one informant is right and the other wrong, but that both perspectives must be considered in assessing the children's functioning. Poor agreement has also been found between DISC diagnoses and clinicians' diagnoses of the same subjects (Costello et al., 1984; Shaffer et al., 1988).

Most experts now agree that data are needed from both children and parents, but no procedures have yet been agreed upon for deciding on categorical diagnoses derived from interviews of different informants (Hodges, 1993). Complex "optimal informant" procedures have been proposed for combining information across multiple sources and diagnoses (Loeber, Green, Lahey, & Stouthamer-Loeber, 1989). However, such procedures appear to have no more psychometric advantages than does a simple combination rule that acknowledges a diagnosis if symptoms are reported by either a child or parent (the "or" rule; Bird, Gould, & Staghezza, 1992; Hodges, 1993; Piacentini, Cohen, & Cohen, 1992). Using the "or" rule to combine child and parent data from the DISC 2.1 produced test-retest kappas ranging from .50 to .71 for five types of diagnoses in a clinical sample. In a community sample, comparable test-retest reliabilities (kappas = .51 to .64) were also obtained with combined parent and child data for attention deficit disorder, oppositional defiant disorder, and conduct disorder. However, reliabilities remained lower for anxiety disorders and depression/dysthymia (kappas = .26 to .32; Jensen et al., 1994).

A problem related to modest parent-child agreement is the heavy reliance on the interview as the primary source of data on children's functioning. Although most experts now acknowledge the need for multiple data sources, "best estimate diagnoses" are still based primarily on interview data (Costello, 1989; Costello et al., 1993). Yet interviews are vulnerable to errors even when questions and response formats are highly structured. For example, Young et al. (1987) listed several sources of potential error and misinformation affecting interviews, including the structure of the interview questions, characteristics of the respondent, and characteristics of the interviewer. Such misinformation is exacerbated when interviews are used to assess problems that might be better assessed in other ways. An example is asking children whether they are restless, fidgety, or have attention problems, rather than assessing these behaviors through direct observations or standardized rating scales obtained from parents and teachers.

APPLICATION OF PSYCHOMETRIC PRINCIPLES TO CHILD INTERVIEWS

The limitations of existing child interviews prompted us to try a different approach. Most structured and semistructured interviews have been targeted on disorders whose existence was taken for granted. The implicit commitment to such disorders dictated that the interviews be designed to detect these disorders. This approach entailed three additional assumptions that have shaped structured and semistructured interviews. One assumption has been that questioning children about each symptom of a disorder would yield accurate yes-or-no reports of whether the symptom was present. A second assumption has been that children could accurately report whether other diagnostic criteria were met, such as the age of onset, duration, and historical co-occurrence of symptoms. A third assumption has been that a child's affirmation of the diagnostic criteria for a particular disorder meant that the child had the disorder. Taken together, these assumptions imply one-to-one relations between children's interview reports of their own behavioral and emotional problems and the presence versus absence of psychiatric disorders.

A Psychometric Perspective

A psychometric perspective provides a different approach to interviews. According to this perspective, interviews involve *measurement* in the same way that tests, observations, and rating forms do. All measurement is vulnerable to variations that are collectively known as *measurement error*. Measurement error is not limited to actual mistakes, but also includes variations that are inherent in the measuring procedure and in the phenomena being measured. Even measurement of variables as simple and straightforward as people's height is subject to numerous sources of variation ("error"). In measuring a person's height, for example, the subject may stand slightly more erect or less erect from one occasion to another. The measuring device may be pressed more or less firmly on the subject's head and may be read from different angles by the people recording the measurements. If a subject is measured on 10 occasions, the obtained heights are likely to vary across the 10 occasions. For example, a man whose "true" height is 183 centimeters might be measured at between 180 centimeters and 186 centimeters on different occasions. Because of measurement variation, it may in fact be impossible to know what his "true" height really is. Repeated measurements of the same variable are often assumed to be normally distributed. The mean of the various measurements of a man's height may therefore be taken as a good estimate of his true height.

Measurement of Behavioral/Emotional Problems. If a simple physical variable such as a person's height can only be approximated via a series of measurement operations, the "measurement" of behavioral/emotional problems from children's interview reports is likely to be even less precise. Even problems that involve fairly clear behaviors, such as stealing or setting fires, are likely to be vulnerable to variations in children's memory of the behavior, their interpretation of what specific behavior should be reported in answer to an interviewer's questions, and their willingness to report the behavior. The way in which an interviewer scores a child's report is also affected by the interviewer's understanding of what the child says and the interviewer's judgment about whether it constitutes a symptomatic problem. Children's reports of emotions such as anxiety and unhappiness are apt to be vulnerable to additional measurement error, especially when the diagnostic criteria require yes-or-no judgments about whether each emotion occurred at a level to be considered symptomatic and whether other criteria are met for onset, frequency, and duration.

Measurement of Disorders. Over and above the measurement of individual symptoms, the measurement of *disorders* raises additional challenges. According to the DSM, a disorder is deemed to be present if all the requisite criteria are met but absent if they are not met. This means that a minor error in the present-versus-absent measurement of even one criterial feature can lead to incorrect "measurement" of a disorder as present versus absent. For example, the DSM-IV criteria for Attention Deficit Hyperactivity Disorder (ADHD) include a list of 9 items under the heading of *Inattention*. To meet the criterion for Inattention, at least 6 of the 9 must have persisted for at least 6 months to a degree that is maladaptive and inconsistent with developmental level (American Psychiatric Association, 1994). For a child who clearly meets 5 of the 9 criteria, an error in judging one of the remaining 4 criteria (e.g., often does not seem to listen when spoken to directly), can determine whether the child incorrectly receives (or fails to receive) the diagnosis of ADHD.

Coping with Measurement Variation

Rather than assuming one-to-one relations between children's interview reports and the presence of symptoms and disorders, the psychometric approach accepts measurement error as an aspect of all assessment, including interviews. As Einhorn (1988) put it, "the acceptance of error can lead to less error" (p. 65). One way of coping with measurement error is by quantifying assessment procedures to avoid requiring present-versus-absent judgments that may obscure variations in the phenomena being measured as well as variations in the measurement procedures themselves. For example, in using interviews to assess child psychopathology, we can quantify each problem that is assessed. We can also quantify the syndrome constructs that are defined by multiple problems. Quantification of this sort can reveal the inevitable measurement variations that would otherwise be camouflaged if we are forced to judge every problem and every syndrome as either present or absent.

A second way of coping with measurement variation is to use multiple items to sample each problem domain. The interview as a whole and its constituent items are thus viewed as samples of behavior rather than as litmus tests that definitively reveal whether particular disorders are present. Because each item is likely to be affected by unique errors of measurement on a particular occasion, aggregation of items that are affected by different errors of measurement can provide a better index of a variable that underlies all of them than can any one item alone. This is because it is difficult to know what portion of a single item's score accurately reflects an underlying variable versus measurement error that is specific to the item or to the occasion on which the item is assessed. Because different errors of measurement affect each item of an aggregated scale, the errors cancel each other out to some extent. As a result, the aggregated scale score is likely to yield a better estimate of the underlying variable's true score than would an estimate based on a single item.

A third way of coping with measurement variation is to compare an individual child's scale scores with the scale scores obtained by relevant reference groups of peers under similar conditions. Rather than assuming *a priori* that a particular score conclusively reveals a disorder, the comparison with reference groups provides a standard against which to judge the individual child as relatively deviant versus nondeviant.

Psychometric Derivation of Syndrome Scales

The psychometric approach is relevant not only to the scoring of items but also to the derivation of syndromes of co-occurring items. Little is known about the true nature of childhood disorders. Interviews should therefore be designed to add new knowledge of childhood behavioral/emotional problems, rather than being designed only to detect assumed disorders that either may not exist or may not be accurately defined by a particular set of diagnostic criteria.

Because the systematic assessment of children's problems via interviews is still in its infancy, we have adopted a psychometric approach to the development of items and scales for our interview. In our approach, called *multiaxial empirically based assessment and taxonomy*, interviews are regarded as one of several useful methods for sampling children's functioning. Like other methods, interviews cannot obtain all the data needed for comprehensive clinical assessments. Also, like other methods, interviews yield a picture of functioning that is constrained by the particular source of data, i.e., the child, and by the means for obtaining data, i.e., a face-to-face session with the child at one point in time. Because interviews can provide only a partial picture of a child's functioning, they are more valuable when coordinated with other methods that sample other aspects of functioning than when used alone. As described later, our model of multiaxial empirically based assessment and taxonomy involves coordination of interview data with data obtained from other sources by other methods.

We designed the SCICA protocol to guide interviewers in eliciting and observing a broad sample of children's behavior in relation to a variety of topics and situations. The

SCICA thus differs from structured interviews that consist mainly of questions whose yes-or-no responses constitute the data obtained from the interview. Instead of being restricted to questions about diagnostic criteria, the SCICA is designed to assess personal style, experiences, and problems that may be unique to particular children, as well as problems and syndromes that are scored in the same standardized fashion across all children.

To develop rating forms for scoring data from the SCICA, we adapted many candidate items for scoring observations and self-reports from our instruments for obtaining reports of children's behavior from parents and teachers, as explained later. Other items were developed specifically for the SCICA. The observation and self-report items have been progressively refined by testing them with different interviewers who used the SCICA with numerous children. Items that were difficult to rate or that never occurred were modified or eliminated. Other items were split apart or lumped together. New items were added to take account of interview responses and observations that were not adequately tapped by the existing items.

To move beyond the level of individual items as molecular samples of behavior, we did statistical analyses of item scores in order to identify sets of problems that tended to co-occur. From these sets of co-occurring problems, we constructed syndrome scales. Each syndrome scale constitutes a quantitative summary of a particular group of co-occurring problems, as sampled by the SCICA. The scores on all the items of a syndrome can be viewed as repeated measurements of the underlying variable that is represented by the syndrome scale. Each item of the syndrome provides a separate way of measuring the variable represented by the scale. Because the items are likely to sample slightly different aspects of functioning and are affected by different measurement errors, their combined scores can more accurately measure the underlying variable than can any single item by itself. Syndrome scores obtained from other assessment procedures can be compared with SCICA syndrome scores to further broaden the sampling of children's functioning.

MULTIAXIAL EMPIRICALLY BASED ASSESSMENT

We developed the SCICA as one component of multiaxial assessment that employs data from multiple sources, including parents, teachers, standardized tests, physical assessments, and direct observations, as well as interviews. To facilitate multiaxial assessment, the SCICA was specifically designed to mesh with data obtained from parent ratings on the Child Behavior Checklist/4-18 (CBCL/4-18; Achenbach, 1991b), teacher ratings on the Teacher's Report Form (TRF; Achenbach, 1991c), direct observations on the Direct Observation Form (DOF; see Achenbach, 1991b), and adolescents' self-ratings on the Youth Self-Report (YSR; Achenbach, 1991d).

The *Integrative Guide for the 1991 CBCL/4-18, YSR, and TRF Profiles* (Achenbach, 1991a) describes our model of multiaxial assessment for the preschool years through adolescence. (Hereafter, we refer to the CBCL/4-18 as the CBCL.) The model includes the following five axes, as summarized in Table 1-1 for ages 6 to 18:

> **Axis I—Parent Data**. Standardized ratings of children's competencies and problems by parents, as on the CBCL; history of the child's development, problems, competencies, and interests as reported by parents in interviews and questionnaires; potential workability of parents for various interventions.

> **Axis II—Teacher Data**. Standardized ratings of the child's school performance and problems by teachers, such as on the TRF; history of the child's school performance as reported by teachers on report cards,

comments in school records, and in teacher interviews; potential workability of teachers for various interventions.

Axis III—Cognitive Assessment. Ability tests, such as the Wechsler Intelligence Scale for Children-Third Edition (WISC-III, Wechsler, 1991) or Kaufman Assessment Battery for Children (KABC; Kaufman & Kaufman, 1983); achievement tests; tests of perceptual-motor skills and speech and language functioning.

Axis IV—Physical Assessment. Height and weight; physical abnormalities and handicaps; medical and neurological examinations; medication history.

Axis V—Direct Assessment of the Child. Standardized clinical interviews, such as the SCICA; direct observations in customary environments such as school, recorded on instruments such as the DOF; standardized self-ratings by adolescents, such as on the YSR; self-concept measures; personality tests; potential workability of the child for various interventions.

The model in Table 1-1 provides guidelines rather than rigid prescriptions that must be precisely followed in all cases. It is not assumed that all sources of data will always be relevant or available for assessment of every child. For example, self-ratings would not be expected for children who are under age 11 or who are not capable of reflecting on their own behavior. In most cases, parent reports are highly relevant, but may not be available from both parents if the child lives with only one parent or a parent surrogate. Teachers' reports are usually relevant for school children if one or more teachers are available to provide them. For most adolescents, self-reports on rating scales are feasible for many of the same problems rated by parents and teachers.

Within the context of the multiaxial model, clinical interviews may be especially useful for assessing children's

Table 1-1

Examples of Multiaxial Assessment Procedures

Approx. Age Range	Axis I Parent Reports	Axis II Teacher Reports	Axis III Cognitive Assessment	Axis IV Physical Assessment	Axis V Direct Assessment of Child
6-12	CBCL/4-18[a] History Parent interview	TRF[b] School records Teacher interview	Ability tests Achievement tests Perceptual-motor tests Language tests	Height, Weight Medical exam Neurological exam	SCICA[c] DOF[d]
13-18	CBCL/4-18 History Parent interview	TRF School records Teacher interview	Ability tests Achievement tests Perceptual-motor tests	Height, Weight Medical exam Neurological exam	SCICA YSR[e] Self-Concept measures Personality tests

[a]CBCL/14-18 = Child Behavior Checklist/4-18 (Achenbach, 1991b)
[b]TRF = Teacher's Report Form (Achenbach, 1991c)
[c]SCICA = Semistructured Clinical Interview for Children and Adolescents (McConaughy & Achenbach, 1994)
[d]DOF = Direct Observation Form (see Achenbach, 1991b)
[e]YSR = Youth Self-Report (Achenbach, 1991d)

views and understanding of their own problems, observing children's behavior and coping strategies, and assessing children's workability for different intervention strategies, such as behavioral programs versus counseling. Data from child interviews can also be combined with data from other sources to derive DSM diagnoses when necessary for clinical or research purposes.

PURPOSE OF THE SCICA

In developing the SCICA, we sought to avoid the limitations imposed by the emphasis on categorical diagnoses that has characterized most previous structured and semistructured interviews. Instead, we employed the psychometric approach used to develop the CBCL, TRF, YSR, and DOF (Achenbach, 1991a, 1993). This involved assessment of many clinically referred children to determine what types of problems were actually observed and reported by children during clinical interviews. Such an approach is not without a conceptual framework, nor is it incompatible with categorical diagnoses like those in the DSM. In fact, several studies have reported significant relations between DSM-III diagnoses and syndromes derived from the CBCL, TRF, and YSR (e.g., Biederman, Faraone, Doyle, Lehman, Kraus, et al., 1993; Edelbrock & Costello, 1988; Mattison & Bagnato, 1987; Rey & Morris-Yates, 1992; Weinstein, Noam, Grimes, Stone, & Schwab-Stone, 1990). However, rather than restricting our interview to DSM diagnoses, we designed the SCICA to function as one component of multiaxial empirically based assessment in the following ways:

1. A semistructured protocol of questions and procedures was developed to sample children's functioning across a variety of topics and tasks.

2. Standardized rating forms were developed for scoring interviewers' observations and children's self-reported problems during the clinical interview.

3. Multiple items on the rating scales were used to sample a broad range of observed and self-reported problems.

4. To facilitate cross-informant comparisons, many SCICA observation and self-report items were drawn from items scored by parents on the CBCL and teachers on the TRF.

5. Statistical procedures were used to aggregate SCICA items into quantitative syndrome scales to measure different problem areas.

6. Standard scores were derived for each syndrome scale, Internalizing, Externalizing, and total problems to indicate how a particular child compares with other children.

7. Tests of reliability and validity were performed on SCICA scores derived from observations and children's self-reports.

8. Scores on the SCICA scales were compared to scores on the CBCL from parents, TRF from teachers, and direct observations obtained with the DOF for the same children.

SUMMARY

Efforts to standardize clinical interviews were prompted by findings of poor agreement among diagnoses made from unstandardized interviews. Structured diagnostic interviews are designed to make particular diagnoses by scoring criterial symptoms as present or absent on the basis of interviewees' reports of each symptom. Semistructured interviews employ more open-ended questions and flexible sequences of topics.

Certain limitations of the existing interviews prompted us to develop the SCICA. The limitations include:

1. The incompatibility of the rigid format of structured interviews with the cognitive levels and interaction styles of preadolescent children.

2. The poor test-retest reliabilities and large declines in self-reported symptoms obtained for preadolescent children over brief intervals.

3. The focus on DSM (or ICD) diagnoses as the main product of the interview.

4. The dichotomous categorization of each child as a case versus noncase with respect to the target diagnoses.

5. The failure to assess important characteristics that are not included among specific diagnostic criteria.

6. The role of the interview as the most salient source of data about the child.

7. The lack of provision for systematically integrating interview data with other types of data about the child.

8. The intricate questioning and scoring that may interfere with rapport and observations.

To overcome these limitations, the SCICA is designed to sample children's functioning in ways that are compatible with their cognitive levels and interaction styles; to yield psychometrically sound scores for observations and self-reports in terms of empirically derived scales; and to provide data that can be meshed with data from other sources in a multiaxial approach to assessment.

Chapter 2
Administration and
Scoring of the SCICA

The SCICA is a standardized semistructured clinical interview for ages 6-18. Although the interview protocol is semistructured, the SCICA is scored quantitatively on structured Observation and Self-Report Forms. The items of the two scoring forms are aggregated into a profile of empirically derived syndrome scales. The SCICA can be administered in approximately 60 to 90 minutes, depending on whether optional sections are included, as described later.

No interview should serve as the sole basis for making diagnoses or other important decisions about children. Instead, the responsible professional will compare interview data with data obtained from other sources for evaluation and treatment decisions. As explained in Chapter 1, the SCICA is designed to mesh with data obtained from parents on the CBCL, teachers on the TRF, and self-reports from adolescents on the YSR. SCICA data should also be integrated with standardized test data, medical data, developmental history, and—when feasible—observations in group settings such as classrooms, using the DOF.

The SCICA should be administered by a professional who is trained in clinically interviewing children and using standardized assessment procedures. User qualifications are described on pages iii and iv. To use the SCICA properly, the interviewer must have sufficient prior experience with children to be comfortable talking with them, to encourage spontaneous responses from them, and to handle the many unexpected events that may occur. The SCICA is designed to be nonstressful, but also to tactfully probe areas that may be sensitive for some children. It is intended to foster a therapeutic alliance in order to maximize the value of assessment and lay the foundations for possible interventions. Because the SCICA is a direct assessment procedure, it is essential to obtain permission from parents or parent surrogates prior to interviewing subjects under age 18.

The SCICA is designed to sample diverse areas of functioning in ways that are geared to the cognitive and emotional levels of the interviewees. The SCICA is not designed to obtain yes/no reports of symptoms. Instead, it utilizes open-ended questions and structured tasks to encourage subjects to talk and behave in ways that will reveal their thoughts, feelings, concerns, and interests, as well as their interaction style in a prototypic mental health assessment situation. The interviewer should follow the standard procedures for administering the SCICA, but should also feel free to tailor questions and probes to the subject's characteristics.

It is usually helpful to have parents complete the CBCL prior to the SCICA. If the subject has school problems, it is also helpful to have a teacher complete the TRF. However, to prevent other data from biasing the SCICA, we recommend that the interviewer know as little as possible about the subject before the interview. An assistant should select six problems scored on the CBCL or TRF and record them on the SCICA Protocol Form prior to the interview. These problems are to be entered in a special section of the protocol where they will not be seen by the interviewer until the last part of the interview. (Details of recording procedures are described later.) In some cases, it may not be possible or appropriate to minimize the interviewer's prior knowledge of the subject. For example, there may be no assistant available to record the CBCL or TRF items, or the interviewer may already be familiar with the subject or may have previously discussed the subject with parents, teachers, or other professionals. In such cases, the interviewer can still obtain a valid assessment with the SCICA by completing and scoring the SCICA before examining the CBCL or TRF scoring profiles and other clinical data. For certain other cases, prior knowledge about the subject may be necessary to assess danger to self or others, suspected abuse, or other referral complaints. In these cases, the interviewer must decide whether the SCICA is appropriate or whether other procedures should be used in conjunction with or in place of the SCICA.

MATERIALS AND GENERAL INSTRUCTIONS

The following materials are needed for administering and scoring the SCICA:

SCICA Protocol Form

SCICA Observation and Self-Report Forms

SCICA Profile (hand- or computer-scored)

Drawing paper and pencil

User-selected standardized tests of mathematics and reading recognition

Soft ball (e.g., nerf ball)

Play materials (blocks; doll family with mother, father, boy, girl, baby, and additional adult and child figures; doll house furniture)

Audio tape recorder (optional)

The interview should be conducted in a private location with only the subject and interviewer present, unless there is a good reason for another person to be present. The interviewer begins by saying:

"We are going to spend some time talking and doing things together, so that I can get to know you and learn about what you like and don't like. This is a private talk. I won't tell your parents or your teachers what you say unless you tell me it is OK. The only thing I might tell is if you said you were going to hurt yourself, hurt someone else, or someone has hurt you."

If the interviewer cannot guarantee confidentiality, the introductory remarks should be altered appropriately. However, it is important to protect the confidentiality of the subject's specific statements, such as those that may be recorded on the SCICA Protocol Form or on tape. If a tape recorder is used, the interviewer can explain this by saying, *"We are going to record our talk on this tape recorder to help remember our time together."* The audiotape should be stored in a safe location and erased after the interviewer has completed all scoring and written reports of the proceedings.

SCICA PROTOCOL FORM

The SCICA Protocol Form, shown in Figure 2-1, outlines the topics, questions, and tasks to be covered in nine broad areas:

1. Activities, school, job

2. Friends

3. Family relations

4. Fantasies

5. Self perception, feelings

6. Parent/teacher-reported problems

7. Achievement tests (optional)

8. For ages 6-12: Screen for fine and gross motor abnormalities (optional)

9. For ages 13-18: Somatic complaints, alcohol, drugs, trouble with the law

Topic areas are organized in a modular fashion. Sections 1 to 6 are intended for all subjects aged 6-18. Sections 1 to 5 should be covered before Sections 6 to 9, but the interviewer can alter the sequence of topics and questions in Sections 1 to 5 to follow the subject's natural flow of conversation. Section 7 is optional for all ages. Section 8 is also optional, but is intended only for ages 6-12. Section 9 is administered last and only to ages 13-18. Administration time for SCICA Sections 1 to 6 is approximately 60 minutes. An additional 20-30 minutes is usually required for Sections 7 and 8 and 5-10 minutes for Section 9 for ages 13-18. Sections 7 and 8 can be omitted to limit the SCICA to one hour, but this provides a less comprehensive assessment of the subject's functioning. Omission of Sections 7 and 8 also sacrifices the opportunity to observe possible differences in behavior and affect during structured tasks versus the open-ended questions and tasks of Sections 1-6.

Play materials should be available for use with young children who are reluctant to engage in conversation or other planned activities. The play materials listed previously are usually sufficient to elicit play activities related to several topic areas of the SCICA Protocol. The subject's play can then provide take-off points for questions, as discussed further in Chapter 3.

The SCICA Protocol Form provides space for recording notes during the interview. The interviewer can use the first column, labeled "Observations," for recording observations of the subject's behavior, affect, and interaction style during the interview. The second column, labeled "Self-Reports," can be used to briefly note the subject's conversation and responses to questions. The interviewer should use these notes as memory aids for scoring the SCICA Observation

SEMISTRUCTURED CLINICAL INTERVIEW FOR CHILDREN AND ADOLESCENTS AGED 6-18
PROTOCOL FORM

					ID#
SUBJECT'S NAME	First	Middle	Last	DATE	INTERVIEWER

The SCICA uses a standard series of topics and tasks to sample functioning in 9 broad areas: 1) Activities, school, job; 2) Friends; 3) Family relations; 4) Fantasies; 5) Self perception, feelings; 6) Parent/teacher-reported problems; 7) Achievement tests (optional); 8) For ages 6-12: Screen for fine and gross motor abnormalities (optional); and 9) For ages 13-18: Somatic complaints, alcohol, drugs, trouble with the law. The interviewer should try to cover all areas appropriate for the subject's age. The sequence of questions and topics in Sections 1-5 may be altered to follow the natural flow of the subject's conversation. The wording should be adapted to the subject's level. For Sections 1-5, open-ended questions and probes are appropriate. Sections 6-9 should be covered after Sections 1-5. An assistant (or, if necessary, the interviewer) should insert six CBCL or TRF problems in Section 6 as instructed on the protocol. The interview should be audio or video taped if possible. Notes regarding the interviewer's observations and subject's self reports can be written in the columns provided. The interviewer should score the subject on the SCICA Observation and Self-Report Form immediately after the interview.

The interviewer begins by saying: *"We are going to spend some time talking and doing things together, so that I can get to know you and learn about what you like and don't like. This is a private talk. I won't tell your parents or your teachers what you say unless you tell me it is OK. The only thing I might tell is if you said you were going to hurt yourself, hurt someone else, or someone has hurt you."* (If a tape recorder is used: *"We are going to record our talk on this tape recorder to help remember our time together."*) The interviewer then addresses the first topic area or other areas initiated by the subject. Play materials can be used with young children who are reluctant to talk or participate in drawing activities. The topics are then addressed by incorporating questions into discussion during play. The following play materials should be available for preadolescents: wooden blocks; doll family with mother, father, boy, girl, baby, and other adult figures; doll house furniture. Specific questions for ages 13-18 are indicated on the protocol.

1. ACTIVITIES, SCHOOL, JOB	OBSERVATIONS	SELF-REPORTS
Activities		
What do you like to do in your spare time, like when you're not in school? Do you participate in any sports/hobbies/clubs?		
What is your favorite TV show/ star/band/TV or story character? What do you like about that show/star/band/character?		
School		
(If age ≥ 16: Do you go to school?)		
What school do you go to? What grade are you in?		
What do you like best in school? What do you like about _____?		
What do you like least in school? What don't you like about _____?		

Figure 2-1. Instructions and questions on Page 1 of the SCICA Protocol Form.

1. ACTIVITIES, SCHOOL, JOB, cont.	OBSERVATIONS	SELF-REPORTS
School, cont. How about your teachers. Which teacher do you like best? What do you like about _____? Which teacher do you like least? What don't you like about _____? How much homework do you have? When do you do your homework? Does anyone help you? Tell me how that works out, having _____ help you. What subjects do you have trouble with? Do you get any special help? Do you ever get in trouble in school? Do you ever worry about school? If you could change something about school, what would it be? **Job (ages 13-18)** Do you have a job? How do you feel about your job/boss? Do you have other ways to earn money? Do you get an allowance?		
2. FRIENDS How many friends do you have? Do you think that is enough friends? Are your friends boys or girls? How old are your friends? What do you do with your friends? Do they come to your house? Do you go to their house? How often? Tell me about someone you like. What do you like about _____? Tell me about someone you don't like. What don't you like about _____?		

Figure 2-1 (cont.). Page 2 of the SCICA Protocol Form.

2. FRIENDS, cont.	OBSERVATIONS	SELF-REPORTS
Do you ever have problems getting along with other kids? What kinds of problems do you have? What do you try to do about _____? Do you ever feel lonely or left out of things? What do you do when that happens? Do you ever get into fights or arguments with other kids? Do the fights involve yelling or hitting? Does that happen with one other kid or with a group? What usually starts the fights? How do they usually end? What are some other ways you could solve that problem, besides fighting? **Additional re: Friends (ages 13-18)** How do you feel about dating/dances/parties? Do you have a girlfriend/boyfriend? How does your family feel about your social life?		
3. FAMILY RELATIONS Who are the people in your family? Who lives in your home? In your home, do the kids have separate rooms? How do you like having separate rooms/sharing a room with _____? Who makes the rules in your home? What happens when kids break the rules? Do you think the rules are fair or unfair? What are the punishments in your home? Who punishes you when you do something wrong? Do you think the punishments are fair or unfair? How do your parents get along? Do they have arguments? (If yes) What are the arguments about? How do you feel when they argue like that? If you could change something in your family or home, what would it be?		

Figure 2-1 (cont.). Page 3 of the SCICA Protocol Form.

3. FAMILY RELATIONS, cont.	OBSERVATIONS	SELF-REPORTS
Kinetic Family Drawing (ages 6-12; optional for ages 13-18) Provide pencil and paper. Ask *S* to **"draw a picture of your family doing something together."** The questions below are asked about the drawing once it is completed. Each family member is discussed. What are they doing? What kind of a person is _____? Tell me three words to describe _____. How does _____ feel in that picture? What is _____ thinking? Who do you get along with best/least? What is going to happen next in your picture? **Description of Family (ages 13-18)** (If no drawing is requested.) Tell me about the people in your family. What kind of a person is _____? Who do you get along with best/least? Does your family set a time for you to be in at night? How do you feel about that?		
4. FANTASIES If you had 3 wishes, what would you wish? Reasons for each? What would you like to be when you're older? If you could change one thing about yourself, what would it be?		
5. SELF PERCEPTION, FEELINGS Tell me a little more about yourself. What makes you happy? What makes you sad? What do you do when you're sad? What makes you mad? What do you do when you're mad? What makes you scared? What do you do when you're scared? What do you worry about? How do you feel most of the time? What do you need the most? Have you had any strange experiences or things happen that you don't understand? (Pursue any indication of suicidal or strange thoughts.)		

Figure 2-1 (cont.). Page 4 of the SCICA Protocol Form.

6. PARENT/TEACHER-REPORTED PROBLEMS	OBSERVATIONS	SELF-REPORTS
Problems are selected from those scored 2 on a CBCL or TRF Profile scale where *S* has a high score, or other problems that are of concern. Six problems are recorded below before the interview. Introduce problems to *S* by saying: *"I want to talk to you about problems kids sometimes have and hear your opinion about them. Some kids have problems with ____. Is that a problem for you?"* 1._____ 2._____ 3._____ 4._____ 5._____ 6._____		
7. ACHIEVEMENT TESTS (Optional) Two user-selected standardized tests are administered. Total time 15-20 minutes. **Mathematics test** **Reading Recognition test**		
8. FOR AGES 6-12: SCREEN FOR FINE & GROSS MOTOR ABNORMALITIES (Optional) **Writing Sample** *S* is asked to write 3 sentences about something *S* likes or to write the alphabet if *S* cannot write sentences. **Gross Motor Screening** *S* is asked to move to the opposite end of the room to **"do some things on left and right and play catch."** Check whether *S* passes each item below. Show right hand ____, left foot ____, left hand ____, right foot ____. Hop on one foot, left ____, right____. Catch ball with two hands ____, right hand ____, left hand ____.		

Figure 2-1 (cont.). Page 5 of the SCICA Protocol Form.

9. FOR AGES 13-18: SOMATIC COMPLAINTS, ALCOHOL, DRUGS, TROUBLE WITH LAW

Subjects aged 13-18 should be questioned directly about the problems listed below. Record responses and use as basis for scoring the items listed on page 5 of the SCICA Self-Report Form. Introduce problems to S by saying: **"Now I want to ask you about some specific types of problems. Over the past 6 months have you had ____? Was there a physical or medical cause for it? How often did you have _____?"**

	Refused	No	Yes	If yes, caused by?	How often? (Probe for <once/mo.; once/wk. to once/mo.; >once/wk.)
228. Aches or pains?	☐	☐	☐	_____
229. Headaches?	☐	☐	☐	_____
230. Nausea, feeling sick?	☐	☐	☐	_____
231. Overeating?	☐	☐	☐	_____
232. Problems with eyes?	☐	☐	☐	_____
233. Rashes, skin problems?	☐	☐	☐	_____
234. Stomachache, cramps?	☐	☐	☐	_____
235. Vomiting, throwing up?	☐	☐	☐	_____
236. Numbness, tingling?	☐	☐	☐	_____
237. Heart pounding?	☐	☐	☐	_____
238. Trouble falling asleep?	☐	☐	☐	_____
239. Waking too early?	☐	☐	☐	_____
240. Other physical problems?	☐	☐	☐	_____

"Now I want to ask you about some other things. Over the past 6 months, have you _____?"

	Refused	No	Yes	Response	If yes, how often? (Probe for <once/mo.; once/wk. to once/mo.; >once/wk.)
241. Drunk beer, wine, or liquor? Been drunk from alcohol?	☐	☐	☐		_____
242. Been stoned or high on drugs?	☐	☐	☐		_____
243. Had strong urge for more drugs?	☐	☐	☐		_____

	Refused	No	Yes	Response	If yes, how often? (Probe for <once/day; 1-5 times/day; >5 times/day)
244. Used tobacco?	☐	☐	☐		_____

	Refused	No	Yes	Response	If yes, how often? (Probe for once; 2-3 times; >3times)
245. Received traffic tickets? (exclude parking)	☐	☐	☐		_____
246. Been in other trouble with the police or law?	☐	☐	☐		_____

Figure 2-1 (cont.). Page 6 of the SCICA Protocol Form.

and Self-Report Forms after the interview is completed. The Observation and Self-Report Forms should be reviewed prior to the interview to familiarize the interviewer with specific behaviors and self-reported problems that are to be scored after the interview. The next sections outline the questions and tasks for each of the nine topic areas of the SCICA Protocol.

1. Activities, School, Job

The interviewer begins by addressing the first topic area on the SCICA Protocol or other topics initiated by the subject. Section 1 contains questions about activities and school for ages 6-18, plus additional questions about jobs for adolescents. Discussion of activities can be used as a "warm-up," prior to questions about school, friends, family, and personal issues. School may represent a sensitive topic area for children experiencing academic difficulties or problems with peers or teachers. If the subject initially seems reluctant to discuss school issues, the interviewer can move to other topic areas and return later to the school questions, after having established rapport with the subject. Questions can also be flexibly sequenced for other topic areas, such as friends, family relations, etc. Questions for Section 1 are listed on pages 1 and 2 of the SCICA Protocol.

2. Friends

Questions for Section 2 listed on pages 2 and 3 are designed to assess the subject's social contacts, relations with friends, and perceptions of peers. Questions concerning problems getting along with other kids, feeling lonely, and fighting or arguing are also intended to assess the subject's social problem-solving skills and coping strategies.

3. Family Relations

Section 3 covers family relations. The interviewer begins with questions listed on page 3 about members of the family and living arrangements. Additional questions assess the subject's relationships with family members, understanding of family rules and punishments, and opinions regarding the fairness of rules and punishments. The subject is also queried regarding perceptions of parental relationships and fantasies about changes in the family or home situation.

To provide an additional mode for discussing family issues, the interviewer obtains a *Kinetic Family Drawing* (KFD). The KFD should be requested from all subjects aged 6-12. The KFD is optional for ages 13-18, but may be useful for adolescents who are reluctant to discuss their family directly. The interviewer introduces the KFD by asking the subject to *"draw a picture of your family doing something together."* After the drawing is completed, the interviewer asks the subject to describe each family member and relations with that member, using the sample questions listed on page 4 of the SCICA Protocol.

The interviewer should record notes on the SCICA Protocol regarding the subject's behavior and responses to questions about the KFD for later scoring of relevant items on the SCICA Observation and Self-Report Forms. For purposes of the SCICA, the KFD is not intended as a projective test, though some users may choose to interpret it projectively for other purposes (see Burns, 1982). If the subject refuses to draw the family, the interviewer should still encourage discussion of the family by asking questions similar to those for the KFD, plus an additional question for ages 13-18 regarding rules for being home at night.

4. Fantasies

Questions in Section 4 (page 4) are designed to sample aspects of children's fantasies or concerns about themselves or their circumstances. For example, asking the subject to express three wishes can tap desires for material objects or basic needs (e.g., big house, food, toys, money) versus more abstract or social concerns (e.g., everyone to be happy, world peace, no pollution). Other questions elicit fantasies about the subject's ideal self and future goals.

5. Self Perception, Feelings

Section 5 (page 4) assesses children's self-perceptions, feelings, worries, and experiences that might be viewed as strange. Initial questions concern what makes the subject happy, sad, mad, and scared. Questions about negative feelings should be followed by probes regarding behavior or social interactions associated with that particular feeling. For example, many children can identify something that makes them mad (e.g., arguing with sister/brother/peer, being denied something, being scolded). To assess responses to angry feelings, the interviewer should then ask the subject, "What do you do when you are mad?" (e.g., throw temper tantrums, hit, sulk, leave the room).

If the subject gives any indication of suicidal thoughts or behavior, the interviewer should probe further to determine the extent of risk, by asking questions about plans, available methods, and suicide attempts. If the subject reports having had strange ideas or experiences, the interviewer should probe further to determine whether these involve delusions, hallucinations, or other possible symptoms of a thought disorder.

6. Parent/Teacher-Reported Problems

Section 6 is designed to assess the subject's perceptions of specific problems reported by parents and/or teachers. Spaces are provided on page 5 of the SCICA Protocol for recording six specific problems reported by parents and/or teachers. Problems should be selected from items that were scored 2 ("very true or often true") by parents on the CBCL and/or teachers on the TRF. The CBCL or TRF items should be selected from syndrome scales showing the highest scores for a particular subject (for scoring of the CBCL and TRF, see Achenbach, 1991b, 1991c). If multiple scales are similarly elevated, the items should be drawn from as many as possible. If possible, the six items should represent a sampling of different problems reported for a particular child, rather than being associated with only one problem area. If fewer than six problems were scored *2*, then items scored *1* can be listed. If parents have reported special concerns about the subject, these problems can be listed along with specific CBCL or TRF items. If neither the CBCL nor TRF have been completed prior to the interview, referral complaints or other reported problems can be addressed in Section 6 in place of CBCL or TRF items.

The parent/teacher-reported problems should be recorded on the SCICA Protocol prior to the interview. As indicated earlier, having an assistant record the items on the SCICA Protocol will minimize the interviewer's prior knowledge of problems reported by parents or teachers. The interviewer should introduce the problems by saying: *"I want to talk to you about problems kids sometimes have and hear your opinion about them. Some kids have problems with_____. Is that a problem for you?"*

The SCICA Protocol provides space for recording the subject's observed behavior and responses to questions about each of the six problems listed.

7. Achievement Tests (Optional)

In Section 7 (page 5), the interviewer administers user-selected standardized mathematics and reading recognition tests. The achievement tests are optional for subjects of all ages, but are particularly recommended for ages 6-12. The tests are intended to sample the subject's cognitive and educational functioning and to assess potential differences in behavior during school-like tasks versus open-ended conversation. The two tests should be administered and scored according to their standard instructions. In our research to develop the SCICA, we used the mathematics and reading recognition subtests of the *Peabody Individual Achievement Test* (PIAT or PIAT-R; Dunn & Markwardt,

1970, 1989). Other standardized mathematics and reading tests can be substituted, such as those of the *Kaufman Test of Educational Achievement* (Kaufman & Kaufman, 1985), *Wechsler Individual Achievement Test* (1992), *Wide Range Achievement Test* (Wilkinson, 1993), or the *Woodcock Johnson Psychoeducational Battery-Revised* (Woodcock & Johnson, 1989). Achievement testing typically takes about 15-20 minutes.

8. For Ages 6-12: Screen for Fine & Gross Motor Abnormalities (Optional)

Section 8 (page 5) includes brief screening tasks for fine and gross motor abnormalities. This section is optional for ages 6-12, and is not used for ages 13-18. The interviewer first obtains a brief writing sample by asking the subject to *"write three sentences about something you like"* or to *"write the alphabet"* if the subject cannot write sentences. To screen for problems in gross motor functioning, the interviewer asks the subject to stand at the opposite end of the room to answer questions about left and right. The interviewer asks the subject to show the right hand, left foot, left hand, right foot, and then to hop first on the left foot and then on the right foot. The SCICA Protocol provides spaces for recording whether the subject passes or fails these screening tasks.

The interviewer then briefly plays catch with the subject using a soft ball, such as a nerf ball. The interviewer should encourage the subject to try catching the ball at least three times with both hands, three times with the right hand, and three times with the left hand. Passes and failures are recorded on the SCICA Protocol. The interviewer can then ask the subject to catch the ball with both hands again or to demonstrate a best throw to end with a positive, easy task.

9. For Ages 13-18: Somatic Complaints, Alcohol, Drugs, Trouble with the Law

Section 9 on page 6 of the SCICA Protocol is used only for ages 13-18. The questions in this section are more structured than those of previous SCICA sections, because adolescents are generally able to give more accurate answers to such structured questions than are preadolescents. The interviewer should record the subject's responses to each question in the spaces provided on the SCICA Protocol. The interviewer should also probe to determine how often each problem has occurred over the preceding 6 months. To assist in later scoring, the questions in Section 9 are numbered 228-246 to correspond to the numbers for the relevant items on page 5 of the SCICA Self-Report Form. The interviewer checks the boxes labeled "refused," "no," or "yes" to record the subject's responses to these items, which are later scored accordingly on the Self-Report Form.

For each somatic complaint reported in questions 228-240, the interviewer should probe to determine whether there was a known physical or medical cause for the problem and note the subject's response on the SCICA Protocol. Additional probes should determine whether the somatic complaint occurred less than once a month, once a week to once a month, or more than once a week.

Questions 241-246 concern use of alcohol, drugs, and tobacco, plus trouble with the law. The interviewer records the subject's response to each question in the spaces provided on the SCICA Protocol. For questions 241-243 concerning problems with alcohol or drugs, the interviewer should probe to determine how often problems have occurred over the past 6 months, similar to probes regarding somatic complaints. For question 244 concerning tobacco use, the interviewer should probe for rates of less than once a day, 1-5 times a day, and more than 5 times a day. For questions 245-246 concerning trouble with the law, the interviewer should probe for rates of once, 2-3 times, and more than 3 times.

Conclusion and Review of Confidentiality

For ages 6-12, Sections 6, 7, or 8 conclude the interview, depending on whether the latter two optional sections are administered. For ages 13-18, Section 9 concludes the interview. After administering the last section, the interviewer briefly summarizes the topics covered and then asks if there is anything else the subject would like to talk about. The interviewer should discuss any new topic the subject brings up.

To end the session, the interviewer thanks the subject for participating and then reviews initial guarantees of confidentiality. The interviewer should inform the subject if a follow-up meeting is planned with parents and/or teachers. The interviewer can then ask the subject for permission to discuss general or specific issues with parents or teachers. We have found that most subjects agree to having the interviewer share their opinions and feelings with important adults. If the subject is reluctant to give such permission, the interviewer should honor the promise of confidentiality, unless problems have been reported that represent a danger to the subject or to others. (As indicated earlier, introductory statements regarding confidentiality specify the exception *"if you were going to hurt yourself, hurt someone else, or someone has hurt you."*) If the subject expresses concerns about confidentiality, the interviewer can usually address important problems or issues with parents or teachers by discussing the relevant items they scored on the CBCL or TRF without referring to specific statements made by the subject during the interview.

SCICA OBSERVATION AND SELF-REPORT FORMS

After the SCICA is completed, the interviewer scores the subject on the SCICA Observation Form, shown in Figure 2-2, and the SCICA Self-Report Form, shown in Figure 2-3.

The Observation Form contains 120 problem items to be scored for ages 6-18, plus an open-ended item (item 121) for recording up to 3 additional problems observed during the interview. The Self-Report Form contains 114 problem items to be scored for ages 6-18, plus an open-ended item (item 247) for recording up to 3 additional problems reported by the subject during the interview. For ages 6-12, items 228-235 cover somatic complaints that are spontaneously reported and scored in the same way as other self-report items. For ages 13-18, items 228-235 for somatic complaints are scored according to the anchor points indicated on page 5. Eleven additional self-report items for ages 13-18 cover other somatic complaints, substance use, and trouble with the law.

It is unnecessary to make a rigorous distinction between what constitutes a subject's self-report versus an observation by the interviewer. Some characteristics qualify for scores on both forms. For example, if a subject reported aggressive exploits that seem implausible or greatly exaggerated, the interviewer may score item *35. Exaggerates or makes up things* on the Observation Form, and item *122. Reports acts of cruelty, bullying or meanness to others, including siblings* on the Self-Report Form. Examples of other items on the Observation Form that may overlap with specific problems scored on the Self-Report Form include: *15. Bragging, boasting*; *17. Can't get mind off certain thoughts; obsessions 52. Lacks self confidence or makes self-deprecating remarks*; *83. Self-conscious or easily embarrassed*; *92. Strange ideas (describe)*; *103. Too fearful or anxious*; and *116. Worries.*

Scoring the SCICA Observation Form

Items on pages 1 and 2 of the SCICA Observation Form describe aspects of the subject's behavior, affect, and interaction style observed during the interview. Each observation item is scored on a 4-point scale according to the following instructions:

SEMISTRUCTURED CLINICAL INTERVIEW--OBSERVATION FORM

ID#

SUBJECT'S FULL NAME	☐ Boy	AGE ____	DATE Mo.____Day____Yr.____	Fa. occup._____
First _____				Mo. occup._____
Middle _____	☐ Girl	GRADE ____	BIRTH Mo.____Day____Yr.____	Interviewer _____
Last _____			ETHNIC GRP. _____	Rater _____

For each item that describes the subject's behavior during the interview, circle: Scoring ages: ☐ 6-12   ☐ 13-18

0 if there was no occurrence

1 if there was a very slight or ambiguous
occurrence

2 if there was a definite occurrence with mild to moderate
intensity and less than 3 minutes duration

3 if there was a definite occurrence with severe intensity or
3 or more minutes duration

The 3-minute duration is a guideline for choosing between ratings of 2 and 3. Italicized numbers and letters to the left of items indicate the scales on which the item is scored. *Score only the item that most specifically describes a particular observation.*

7-0 1 2 3   1. Acts overly confident

  0 1 2 3   2. Acts seductively (describe)_____

7-0 1 2 3   3. Giggles too much

6-0 1 2 3   4. Acts too young for age

4-0 1 2 3   5. Apathetic or unmotivated

8-0 1 2 3   6. Argues

8-0 1 2 3   7. Asks for feedback on performance (describe)

  0 1 2 3   8. Attempts to leave room for reasons other
than toilet

4-0 1 2 3   9. Avoids eye contact

8-0 1 2 3   10. Irresponsible, destructive, or dangerous
behavior (describe)_____

  0 1 2 3   11. Behaves like opposite sex

  0 1 2 3   12. Bites fingernails

  0 1 2 3   13. Bizarre or unusual language (e.g., echolalia,
babbling, nonsense words, neologisms;
describe)_____

8-0 1 2 3   14. Blames difficulty on task or interviewer

7-0 1 2 3   15. Bragging, boasting

7-0 1 2 3   16. Burps or farts without apology

7-0 1 2 3   17. Can't get mind off certain thoughts; obsessions (describe)_____

7-0 1 2 3   18. Chews or sucks on clothing

  0 1 2 3   19. Complains of being bored by interview or
tests

  0 1 2 3   20. Complains of dizziness, headaches or other
somatic problems during session (describe)

8-0 1 2 3   21. Complains of tasks being too hard or upset
by tasks

6-0 1 2 3   22. Concrete thinking

2-0 1 2 3   23. Confused or seems to be in a fog

6-0 1 2 3   24. Contradicts or reverses own statements

  0 1 2 3   25. Cries

7-0 1 2 3   26. Day-dreams or gets lost in thoughts

8-0 1 2 3   27. Defiant, talks back, or sarcastic

8-0 1 2 3   28. Demands must be met immediately

2-0 1 2 3   29. Difficulty following directions

7-0 1 2 3   30. Disjointed or tangential conversation

6-0 1 2 3   31. Doesn't concentrate or pay attention for
long on tasks, questions, topics

6-0 1 2 3   32. Doesn't sit still, restless, or hyperactive

6-0 1 2 3   33. Easily distracted by external stimuli

  0 1 2 3   34. Erases or crosses out a lot in writing or
drawing

7-0 1 2 3   35. Exaggerates or makes up things

8-0 1 2 3   36. Explosive and unpredictable behavior

  0 1 2 3   37. Feels too guilty

6-0 1 2 3   38. Fidgets

  0 1 2 3   39. Fine motor difficulty (describe)_____

8-0 1 2 3   40. Frequently off-task

7-0 1 2 3   41. Gives long, complex verbal responses

6-0 1 2 3   42. Gross motor difficulty or clumsy

8-0 1 2 3   43. Guesses a lot; does not think out
answers or strategies

2-0 1 2 3   44. Has difficulty expressing self verbally
(describe)_____

6-0 1 2 3   45. Has difficulty understanding language
(describe)_____

2-0 1 2 3   46. Has problems remembering facts or
details

  0 1 2 3   47. Hears things that aren't there during
session (describe)_____

8-0 1 2 3   48. Impatient

8-0 1 2 3   49. Impulsive or acts without thinking

2-0 1 2 3   50. Is afraid of making mistakes

Figure 2-2. Instructions and problem items 1-50 of the SCICA Observation Form.

0 = no occurrence
1 = very slight or ambiguous occurrence

2 = mild to moderate intensity and < 3 minutes
3 = severe intensity or ≥ 3 minutes

7-0 1 2 3   51. Jokes inappropriately or too much
2-0 1 2 3   52. Lacks self confidence or makes self-deprecating remarks
6-0 1 2 3   53. Lapses in attention
0 1 2 3   54. Laughs inappropriately
7-0 1 2 3   55. Leaves room during session to go to toilet
4-0 1 2 3   56. Limited conversation
4-0 1 2 3   57. Limited fantasy or imagination
0 1 2 3   58. Lying or cheating
8-0 1 2 3   59. Makes odd noises
8-0 1 2 3   60. Messy work
8-0 1 2 3   61. Misbehaves, taunts, or tests the limits
0 1 2 3   62. Mouth movements while writing or drawing
4-0 1 2 3   63. Needs coaxing
6-0 1 2 3   64. Needs repetition of instructions or questions
2-0 1 2 3   65. Nervous, highstrung, or tense
6-0 1 2 3   66. Nervous movements, twitching, tics, or other unusual movements (describe)_____
6-0 1 2 3   67. Out of seat
2-0 1 2 3   68. Overly anxious to please
0 1 2 3   69. Perseverates on a topic
0 1 2 3   70. Picks or scratches nose, skin, or other parts of body (describe)_____
7-0 1 2 3   71. Plays with own sex parts
4-0 1 2 3   72. Refuses to talk
4-0 1 2 3   73. Reluctant to discuss feelings or personal issues
4-0 1 2 3   74. Reluctant to guess
7-0 1 2 3   75. Repeats certain acts over and over; compulsions (describe)_____
8-0 1 2 3   76. Resistant or refuses to comply (describe)_____
4-0 1 2 3   77. Says "don't know" a lot
8-0 1 2 3   78. Screams
4-0 1 2 3   79. Secretive, keeps things to self
4-0 1 2 3   80. Seems overtired or fatigued
0 1 2 3   81. Seems too dependent on interviewer
4-0 1 2 3   82. Seems unresponsive to humor
2-0 1 2 3   83. Self-conscious or easily embarrassed
8-0 1 2 3   84. Shows off, clowns, or acts silly
4-0 1 2 3   85. Shy or timid
4-0 1 2 3   86. Slow to respond verbally
4-0 1 2 3   87. Slow to warm up

6-0 1 2 3   88. Speech problem (describe)_____
4-0 1 2 3   89. Stares blankly
0 1 2 3   90. Stares intensely at interviewer
7-0 1 2 3   91. Strange behavior (describe)_____
7-0 1 2 3   92. Strange ideas (describe)_____
4-0 1 2 3   93. Stubborn, sullen, or irritable
0 1 2 3   94. Sucks fingers or thumb
8-0 1 2 3   95. Sudden changes in mood or feelings
0 1 2 3   96. Sulks
8-0 1 2 3   97. Suspicious
7-0 1 2 3   98. Swearing or obscene language
8-0 1 2 3   99. Talks aloud to self
7-0 1 2 3   100. Talks too much
8-0 1 2 3   101. Temper tantrums, hot temper, or seems angry
2-0 1 2 3   102. Too concerned with neatness, cleanliness, or order
2-0 1 2 3   103. Too fearful or anxious
2-0 1 2 3   104. Tremors in hands or fingers
8-0 1 2 3   105. Tries to control or manipulate interviewer
4-0 1 2 3   106. Underactive or slow moving
4-0 1 2 3   107. Unhappy, sad, or depressed
0 1 2 3   108. Unusual pitch or tone of voice
0 1 2 3   109. Unusually changeable behavior
8-0 1 2 3   110. Unusually loud
4-0 1 2 3   111. Unusually quiet voice
8-0 1 2 3   112. Wants to quit or does quit tasks
0 1 2 3   113. Whines
4-0 1 2 3   114. Withdrawn, doesn't get involved with interviewer
8-0 1 2 3   115. Works quickly and carelessly
0 1 2 3   116. Worries
0 1 2 3   117. Yawns
0 1 2 3   118. Denies responsibility or blames others
0 1 2 3   119. Flat affect
0 1 2 3   120. Overly dramatic
  121. Add observed problems or behaviors not already listed:
0 1 2 3   _____
0 1 2 3   _____
0 1 2 3   _____

Figure 2-2 (cont.). Problem items 51-121 of the SCICA Observation Form.

SEMISTRUCTURED CLINICAL INTERVIEW--SELF-REPORT FORM

| ID# |

For each item that describes the subject's conversation during the session, circle:

   0 **if there was no occurrence**

   1 **if there was a very slight or ambiguous**
      occurrence

   2 **if there was a definite occurence with mild to moderate**
     intensity and less than 3 minutes duration

   3 **if there was a definite occurrence with severe intensity or**
     3 or more minutes duration

The interview includes "Parent/Teacher-Reported Problems," where the interviewer asks the subject his/her view of 6 problems scored *2* by the parents/teachers on the CBCL/TRF. Score an item *1* if a subject's *only* mention of a problem is to acknowledge the CBCL/TRF report of it without further elaboration. *Score only the item that most specifically describes a particular self-report. Do not score self-reported problems that clearly ended more than 6 months prior to the interview.*

5-0 1 2 3   122. Reports acts of cruelty, bullying or meanness to others, including siblings

  0 1 2 3   123. Reports arguing or fighting with siblings

  0 1 2 3   124. Reports arguing or verbal altercations (except with siblings)

  0 1 2 3   125. Reports behaving like opposite sex

  0 1 2 3   126. Reports being beaten up by others including siblings (exclude parents)

  0 1 2 3   127. Reports being bored in situations other than current interview

1-0 1 2 3   128. Reports being confused or in a fog

  0 1 2 3   129. Reports being cruel to animals

5-0 1 2 3   130. Reports being disobedient at home

5-0 1 2 3   131. Reports being disobedient at school

5-0 1 2 3   132. Reports being impulsive or acting without thinking

  0 1 2 3   133. Reports being jealous of others (describe) _____

1-0 1 2 3   134. Reports being lonely or left out of others' activities

3-0 1 2 3   135. Reports being physically harmed by parent or guardian (describe)_____ _____

3-0 1 2 3   136. Reports being punished a lot at home, including spanking (describe)_____ _____ _____

1-0 1 2 3   137. Reports being self-conscious or easily embarrassed

  0 1 2 3   138. Reports being sexually abused (describe) _____

  0 1 2 3   139. Reports being shy or timid

5-0 1 2 3   140. Reports being suspicious

1-0 1 2 3   141. Reports being too fearful or anxious

3-0 1 2 3   142. Reports being treated unfairly at home

3-0 1 2 3   143. Reports being treated unfairly at school

1-0 1 2 3   144. Reports being unable to concentrate or pay attention for long

5-0 1 2 3   145. Reports being unable to sit still, being restless, or hyperactive

1-0 1 2 3   146. Reports being underactive, slow, or lacking energy

1-0 1 2 3   147. Reports being unhappy, sad, or depressed

  0 1 2 3   148. Reports bowel movements outside toilet

  0 1 2 3   149. Reports compulsive acts (describe) _____

  0 1 2 3   150. Reports concerns about family problems (describe)_____

3-0 1 2 3   151. Reports concerns with neatness or cleanliness

  0 1 2 3   152. Reports crying a lot

  0 1 2 3   153. Reports daydreaming or getting lost in thoughts

  0 1 2 3   154. Reports deliberately harming self or attempting suicide

5-0 1 2 3   155. Reports destroying own property

5-0 1 2 3   156. Reports destroying property belonging to others (exclude vandalism)

1-0 1 2 3   157. Reports difficulty following directions in school or work

1-0 1 2 3   158. Reports difficulty learning

  0 1 2 3   159. Reports disliking school or work

1-0 1 2 3   160. Reports fear of making mistakes

  0 1 2 3   161. Reports fearing he/she might think or do something bad

1-0 1 2 3   162. Reports fears of certain people, animals, situations, or places other than school (describe)_____

  0 1 2 3   163. Reports fears of going to school

1-0 1 2 3   164. Reports feeling guilty

  0 1 2 3   165. Reports feeling he/she must be perfect

  0 1 2 3   166. Reports feeling hurt when criticized

  0 1 2 3   167. Reports feeling nervous or tense

1-0 1 2 3   168. Reports feeling others are out to get him/her

1-0 1 2 3   169. Reports feeling overtired

  0 1 2 3   170. Reports feeling that no one loves him/her

1-0 1 2 3   171. Reports feeling worthless or inferior

  0 1 2 3   172. Reports getting hurt a lot, being accident-prone

5-0 1 2 3   173. Reports getting into physical fights (except with siblings)

Figure 2-3. Instructions and problem items 122-173 of the SCICA Self-Report Form.

0 = no occurrence
1 = very slight or ambiguous occurrence

2 = mild to moderate intensity and < 3 minutes
3 = severe intensity or ≥ 3 minutes

_1_-0 1 2 3   174. Reports getting teased or picked on, including by siblings

_5_-0 1 2 3   175. Reports hanging around others who get into trouble

0 1 2 3   176. Reports hating or disliking brother or sister

_3_-0 1 2 3   177. Reports hating or disliking mother or father

_5_-0 1 2 3   178. Reports hating or disliking teacher, principal or boss

_1_-0 1 2 3   179. Reports having nightmares

0 1 2 3   180. Reports hearing things that aren't there during times other than interview (describe)_____

_3_-0 1 2 3   181. Reports lack of attention from parents, excluding neglect (describe)_____

_5_-0 1 2 3   182. Reports lacking guilt after misbehaving

0 1 2 3   183. Reports lying or cheating

0 1 2 3   184. Reports neglect of basic needs by parent or guardian (describe)_____

_1_-0 1 2 3   185. Reports not being liked by peers

_3_-0 1 2 3   186. Reports not getting along with mother or father

0 1 2 3   187. Reports obsessive thoughts (describe)___

_5_-0 1 2 3   188. Reports physically attacking people, including siblings

0 1 2 3   189. Reports preferring kids older than self

0 1 2 3   190. Reports preferring to be alone

0 1 2 3   191. Reports preferring kids younger than self

_1_-0 1 2 3   192. Reports problems getting along with peers

_1_-0 1 2 3   193. Reports problems making or keeping friends

_1_-0 1 2 3   194. Reports problems with school work or job (describe)_____

0 1 2 3   195. Reports running away from home

_3_-0 1 2 3   196. Reports screaming

0 1 2 3   197. Reports seeing things that aren't there during times other than interview (describe)_____

0 1 2 3   198. Reports setting fires

0 1 2 3   199. Reports showing off or clowning

0 1 2 3   200. Reports stealing at home

0 1 2 3   201. Reports stealing outside of home

0 1 2 3   202. Reports storing up things he/she doesn't need (describe)_____

0 1 2 3   203. Reports sudden changes in mood or feelings

0 1 2 3   204. Reports teasing others, including siblings

_5_-0 1 2 3   205. Reports temper tantrums or hot temper

0 1 2 3   206. Reports thinking about sex a lot

_5_-0 1 2 3   207. Reports threatening other people

0 1 2 3   208. Reports trouble sleeping (describe)
_____

0 1 2 3   209. Reports truancy, skipping school or job

0 1 2 3   210. Reports vandalism

0 1 2 3   211. Reports wetting bed

0 1 2 3   212. Reports wetting self during day

0 1 2 3   213. Reports wishing to be of the opposite sex

_1_-0 1 2 3   214. Reports worrying (describe)_____

0 1 2 3   215. Talks about death, including deaths of animals, family members, etc. (describe)

0 1 2 3   216. Talks about deliberately harming self or attempting suicide (without actually doing so)

0 1 2 3   217. Reports sexual problems or excessive activity (describe)_____

0 1 2 3   218. Talks about physically attacking, hurting, or killing people, including siblings (without actually doing so)

0 1 2 3   219. Talks about war or generalized violence (describe)_____

0 1 2 3   220. Talks about getting revenge without physical attack

0 1 2 3   221. Reports being mad or angry

0 1 2 3   222. Reports strange behavior

0 1 2 3   223. Reports conflict with family re: plans for work or education

0 1 2 3   224. Reports conflict with family re: social activities

0 1 2 3   225. Reports problems in sexual identity or concern about homosexuality

0 1 2 3   226. Reports problems in social relations with opposite sex

0 1 2 3   227. Reports alcohol/drug use without parental permission (describe)_____

FOR AGES 6-12:
Score somatic items only if no known physical cause

0 1 2 3   228. Reports aches or pains in body

_3_-0 1 2 3   229. Reports headaches

0 1 2 3   230. Reports nausea, feeling sick

0 1 2 3   231. Reports overeating

0 1 2 3   232. Reports problems with eyes

0 1 2 3   233. Reports rashes, skin problems

_3_-0 1 2 3   234. Reports stomachache, cramps

0 1 2 3   235. Reports vomiting, throwing up

Go to page 5 for item 247.

Figure 2-3 (cont.). Problem items 174-227, plus items 228-235 scored for ages 6-12, of the SCICA Self-Report Form.

FOR AGES 13-18:
Score somatic items 228-240 only if no known physical cause.
Use the following definitions for scoring items 228-246:

No	Less than once/mo.	Once/wk. to once/mo.	More than once/wk.	Item refused	
0	1	2	3	4	228. Reports aches or pains in body
0	1	2	3	4	229. Reports headaches
0	1	2	3	4	230. Reports nausea, feeling sick
0	1	2	3	4	231. Reports overeating
0	1	2	3	4	232. Reports problems with eyes
0	1	2	3	4	233. Reports rashes, skin problems
0	1	2	3	4	234. Reports stomachache, cramps
0	1	2	3	4	235. Reports vomiting, throwing up
0	1	2	3	4	236. Reports numbness, tingling
0	1	2	3	4	237. Reports heart pounding
0	1	2	3	4	238. Reports trouble falling asleep
0	1	2	3	4	239. Reports waking too early
0	1	2	3	4	240. Reports other physical problems
0	1	2	3	4	241. Reports getting drunk on alcohol within last 6 months
0	1	2	3	4	242. Reports getting stoned or high on drugs within last 6 months
0	1	2	3	4	243. Reports strong urge for more drugs

No	Less than once/day	One to 5 times/day	More than 5 times/day	Item refused	
0	1	2	3	4	244. Reports using tobacco

No	Once	2-3 times	More than 3 times	Item refused	
0	1	2	3	4	245. Reports traffic tickets (exclude parking)
0	1	2	3	4	246. Reports trouble with police/law other than traffic tickets

FOR ALL AGES: Score item 247 according to initial criteria.

247. Add other reported problems not already listed.

0 1 2 3 _____

0 1 2 3 _____

0 1 2 3 _____

Describe any problems that may be important, but fail to meet SCICA scoring criteria, e.g., abuse, firesetting, or suicidal behavior that occurred >6 months ago, using back page if necessary.

Figure 2-3 (cont.). Problem items 228-246 scored for ages 13-18, plus item 247, of the SCICA Self-Report Form.

For each item that describes the subject's behavior during the interview, circle:

0 if there was no occurrence;

1 if there was a very slight or ambiguous occurrence;

2 if there was a definite occurrence with mild to moderate intensity and less than 3 minutes duration; and

3 if there was a definite occurrence with severe intensity or 3 or more minutes duration.

Scoring the SCICA Self-Report Form

Most of the SCICA self-report items were adapted from items on the CBCL and TRF that describe problems a subject might report during an interview. Examples are *122. Reports acts of cruelty, bullying or meanness to others, including siblings*; 130. *Reports being disobedient at home*; and *171. Reports feeling worthless or inferior.* Additional items were developed from subjects' responses during our research on the SCICA. Examples are *127. Reports being bored in situations other than current interview*; *142. Reports being treated unfairly at home*; *181. Reports lack of attention from parents*; and *215. Talks about death, including deaths of animals, family members, etc.* Certain items begin with the phrase "Talks about" because they describe the subject's conversation without indicating that the subject reported their actual occurrence.

Self-report items 122-235 on pages 3 and 4 of the SCICA Self-Report Form are scored on the same 4-point scale used for scoring the observation items. Items 122-227 are scored for all ages. For ages 6-12, items 228-235 on page 4 of the SCICA Self-Report Form describe somatic complaints that are scored according to the same criteria as used for other items. For ages 13-18, items 228-246 on page 5 are scored according to the specific anchor points designated for choosing between ratings of *1*, *2*, and *3*; if a subject refuses to answer a question, score the item *4* to indicate refusal. The numbering of items 228-246 for ages 13-18 corresponds to questions listed in Section 9 on page 6 of the SCICA Protocol. Additional self-reported problems not covered by items 122-246 should be recorded in the spaces under item 247 and scored according to the criteria for items 122-227. Space is also provided on page 5 for recording important problems reported during the interview that do not meet the SCICA scoring criteria. Examples include abuse, fire setting, or suicidal behavior that occurred more than 6 months prior to the interview.

Appendix A provides guidelines for deciding between different observation and self-report items, and for choosing between scores of *1*, *2*, and *3* for specific items.

Summary Notes

Page 6 of the SCICA Observation and Self-Report Forms (not shown in figures) provides space for writing summary notes regarding observations, self-reported problems, and clinical impressions of the subject. The interviewer can use this space to integrate clinical information gathered from the interview and scoring procedures. The summary can also include questions to be answered from other sources, plus hypotheses about the subject's problems and potential treatment options.

SCICA PROFILE FOR AGES 6-12

To enable users to compare a subject's scores with those obtained by other clinically referred subjects, we constructed the SCICA Profile for Ages 6-12, shown in Figure 2-4. The profile is modeled on profiles previously constructed for the CBCL, TRF, and YSR. The profile consists of eight syndrome scales and two broad groupings of Internalizing and Externalizing problems derived from ratings of the 168 clinically referred subjects. Interviews were videotaped for each subject and rated by an observer of the videotape as

SCICA Profile for Ages 6-12

Name _____

Internalizing   Externalizing   Clin T

ID#

Sex: M   F

Age

Date

TOT OB

OB T

TOT SR

SR T

Computations

Scale 1.

+2.

INT

INT T

Scale 5.

6.

7.

+8.

EXT

EXT T

OB Observation Form
SR Self-Report Form

Clin T scale: 100, 95, 90, 85, 80, 75, 70, 65, 60, 55, 50, 45, 40

Clin %ile: 93, 84, 69, 50, 31, 16

Normal Range

1
ANX/DEP SR
128. Confused
134. Lonely
137. SelfConsc
137. DiffDirect
141. Fearful
145. NoConfidence
146. Underactive
147. Sad
157. DiffDirect
158. DiffLearning
160. FearMistakes
162. Fears
164. Guilty
169. Overtired
171. Worthless
174. Teased
185. NotLiked
192. NotGetAlong
193. NoFriends
194. SchoolWork
214. Worries
TOTAL

2
ANXIOUS OB
23. Confused
29. DiffDirect
44. DiffExpress
46. NoRemember
50. FearMistakes
52. NoConfidence
65. Nervous
68. AnxPlease
83. SelfConsc
102. TooNeat
103. Fearful
104. Tremors
TOTAL

3
FAM PROB SR
136. HarmedPar
138. Punished
142. UnfairHome
143. UnfairSchool
151. TooNeat
177. HatesPar
181. NoAttention
186. NotGetAlongPar
196. Screams
229. Headaches
234. Stomachaches
TOTAL

4
WITHDRAWN OB
5. Apathetic
9. AvoidsEye
56. NoConvers
57. NoFantasy
63. NeedsCoax
72. WontTalk
73. WontTalkFeel
74. WontGuess
77. DoontKnow
79. Secretive
80. Overtired
82. NoHumor
85. Shy
86. SlowWarmUp
87. SlowVerbal
89. Stares
93. Stubborn
106. Underactive
107. Sad
111. Quiet
114. Withdrawn
TOTAL

5
AGG BEH SR
122. Mean
130. DiscbHome
131. DiscbSchool
132. Impulsive
140. Suspicious
145. Can'tSitStill
155. DestroysOwn
156. DestroysOthr
175. Bad Compan
178. HatesTeacher
182. NoGuilt
188. Attacks
205. Temper
207. Threatens
TOTAL

6
ATT PROB OB
4. ActsYoung
22. Concrete
24. Reverses
31. Doesn'tConcentrate
32. Doesn'tSitStill
33. Distracted
38. Fidgets
42. Clumsy
45. NotUnderstand
53. Lapses
64. NeedsRepeat
66. Twitches
67. PlaysSelfPart
88. SpeechProb
TOTAL

7
STRANGE OB
1. OverConfident
3. Giggles
15. Brags
16. BurstFants
17. MindOff
18. ChewsCloth
26. Daydreams
30. DisonftConver
35. DemandsMet
41. LongResponses
51. Jokes
55. LeaveToilet
71. PlaysSadPart
75. RepeatsActs
91. StrangeBehav
92. StrangeIdeas
98. TalksMuch
100. TalksMuch
TOTAL

8
RESISTANT OB
6. Argues
7. AsksFeedback
10. Irresolvable
14. BlamesInattnr
21. ComplainsHard
27. Defiant
28. DemandsMet
36. Explosive
40. OffTask
43. Guesses
48. Impatient
49. Impulsive
59. OddNoises
60. MessyWork
61. Mistakshaves
76. Resistant
78. Screams
84. ShowsOff
95. MoodChange
97. Suspicious
99. TalksSelf
101. TamperAngry
105. Manipulates
110. Loud
112. Quits
115. Careless
TOTAL

UNAUTHORIZED COPYING IS ILLEGAL

Figure 2-4. Hand-scored version of the SCICA Profile for Ages 6-12. *T* score tables are omitted from right-hand side of profile. (Computer-scored versions of the profile are shown in Chapter 10.)

well as by the interviewer.   Ratings of each item by the interviewer and the videotape observer were averaged and submitted to principal components analysis to derive sets of items that co-occurred to form syndromes.   We averaged interviewer and observer ratings in order to increase the reliability of scores and to reduce the effects of including interviewers and raters who provided scores for multiple subjects.   After deriving syndrome scales, we performed a principal factor analysis on the correlations among these scales in order to identify groupings of scales that tend to be mutually associated.   Chapter 4 describes characteristics of the research sample and statistical analyses used to develop the SCICA Profile for Ages 6-12.

The eight syndrome scales of the SCICA Profile are: *Aggressive Behavior,*[SR] *Anxious,*[OB] *Anxious/Depressed,*[SR] *Attention Problems,*[OB] *Family Problems,*[SR] *Resistant,*[OB] *Strange,*[OB] and *Withdrawn.*[OB]   The superscript next to the scale name indicates whether the scale was derived from the Observation Form (OB) or the Self-Report Form (SR).   For each syndrome, the profile lists in numerical order the items found to occur together in ratings of our clinical sample. The items listed on the profile are abbreviated versions of those on the SCICA Observation and Self-Report Forms. The syndrome scales are arranged on the profile according to their loadings on the second-order factors derived from the correlations among the syndrome scales.   The two groupings of syndromes identified by the second-order factors are designated as Internalizing and Externalizing. The left end of the profile starts with the Anxious/Depressed syndrome which had the highest loading on the Internalizing factor. This is followed by the Anxious syndrome which had the next highest loading on the Internalizing factor. The two syndromes that did not have high loadings on either Internalizing or Externalizing are listed in the middle of the profile.   The four syndromes with high loadings on the Externalizing factor are listed on the right side of the profile,

ending with Resistant which had the highest loading on the
Externalizing factor.

Scoring the SCICA Profile for Ages 6-12

The interviewer's ratings are entered on the SCICA
Profile to obtain raw scores, T scores, and percentiles for the
eight SCICA syndrome scales. T score equivalents are also
provided for Internalizing and Externalizing, plus total scores
that are computed separately for the Observation and Self-
Report Forms. The SCICA Profile can be scored by hand
or computer. Chapter 4 provides details of the derivation
of percentiles and T scores, based on a sample of 237
clinically referred subjects aged 6-12.

Syndrome Scale Scores. To compute scores on the
syndrome scales, the rater's score (0, 1, 2, 3) for each item
is entered in the space beside the item on the profile. The
italicized numbers to the left of each item on the Observation
and Self-Report Forms indicate the scales on which the items
are scored. The scores for all the items are summed to
obtain the total raw score for each scale. After obtaining the
total raw score for each scale, the user marks the raw scale
scores in the columns on the graphic display to form a
profile depicting the subject's overall pattern of problems.
The computer scoring program automatically assigns the item
scores to scales, computes scale scores, and marks the scale
scores on the profile. Percentiles based on our research
sample can be read from the left side of the graphic display.
T scores based on the same sample can be read from the
right side.

Total Problem Scores. Total problem scores are
computed separately for the Observation Form and Self-
Report Form. The hand-scored SCICA Profile provides
spaces to the right of the graphic display for entering total
raw scores and T scores for the Observation Form (*TOT OB*)

and for the Self-Report Form (*TOT SR*). For ages 6-12, raw scores for total problems on the Observation Form are the sum of the *1*s, *2*s, and *3*s scored on items 1-120. If additional problems have been written in for item 121 on the Observation Form, only the problem with the highest score is counted toward the total score. Raw scores for total problems on the Self-Report Form are the sum of the *1*s, *2*s, and *3*s scored on items 122-235, plus the highest score for any additional problems written in for item 247. The additional problems for items 121 and 247 are scored only if they are not covered more specifically by other SCICA items. The two boxed columns labeled *TOT OB* and *TOT SR* at the far right side of the hand-scored SCICA Profile show the *T* scores corresponding to the raw scores for total problems for the Observation and Self-Report Forms. Total raw scores and *T* scores for the Observation and Self-Report Forms are automatically computed and listed at the top of a column to the right of the SCICA Profile on the computer-scored version.

Internalizing and Externalizing Scores. Raw scores and *T* scores for Internalizing and Externalizing are entered in the spaces provided below the total problem scores on the hand-scored profile. To compute the Internalizing score, the user sums the scores from the two Internalizing syndromes. Externalizing scores are computed in the same way by summing the scores from the four Externalizing syndromes. Space is provided on the hand-scored profile for making these computations. The two boxed columns labeled *INT* and *EXT* to the right of the graphic display on the SCICA Profile show the raw scores and their corresponding *T* scores for Internalizing and Externalizing. The user can mark the number in the column labeled *Raw* that corresponds to the obtained total raw score for Internalizing or Externalizing and then locate its corresponding *T* score in the column to the right labeled *T*. The computer scoring program automatically computes total raw scores and *T* scores for Internalizing and Externalizing and lists them below the total problem scores on the right side of the profile.

Other Problems. In the principal components analyses from which we derived the SCICA syndrome scales, we excluded low prevalence items that were scored as present for <5% of the research sample. We also excluded from the syndrome scales items that had loadings <.30 on rotated components retained from our principal components analyses. As a result, 30 items from the Observation Form and 67 items from the Self-Report Form are not included in the syndrome scales. These remaining items are listed on the back of the hand-scored SCICA Profile, where their scores can be entered in the spaces provided. This step is optional, but is useful for displaying each item's score. The fact that the items were rare or did not have high loadings on a syndrome does not mean that they are unimportant. It simply means that they did not help to discriminate statistically among the empirically derived syndromes. All of the SCICA items are included in the total scores for the Observation Form and Self-Report Form.

Scores for Ages 13-18

There is currently no separate SCICA Profile for ages 13-18, because our scales for adolescents are still being developed. However, items 236-246 for ages 13-18 are listed on the back of the hand-scored SCICA Profile, along with the Other Problems for ages 6-12 discussed above. Users can enter scores for the adolescent items in the spaces provided. The computer-scoring program allows users to enter items 228-246 for ages 13-18, but the profile printout will display a warning that the subject is outside the 6-12 age range. With this caveat in mind, users can obtain scores for adolescents on the SCICA scales currently available for ages 6-12. We will report our findings for ages 13-18 in future publications.

MEANS AND STANDARD DEVIATIONS
ON SCICA SCALES

There are no clinical cutpoints for the SCICA scales, as there are for the CBCL, TRF, and YSR scales (see Achenbach, 1991b, 1991c, 1991d). This is because the SCICA *T* scores are based on a *clinically referred sample* rather than a normative sample like those used to derive *T* scores for the CBCL, TRF, and YSR profiles. Because SCICA *T* scores are based on a clinical sample, they are not intended to indicate the deviance of a subject's behavior from that of nonreferred "normal" subjects.

Appendix C lists means and standard deviations for SCICA scores obtained by matched samples of 53 referred and 53 nonreferred subjects aged 6-12. Users can compare these scores from the referred and nonreferred samples to scores obtained by individual subjects and scores obtained by other samples.

The pattern of high and low scores on the SCICA Profile can be compared to the overall pattern of scores obtained on similar scales of the CBCL and TRF profiles. Such comparisons can highlight similarities and differences in the types of problems exhibited during the clinical interview and in reports by parents and teachers. SCICA scores can also be compared to scores on similar scales of the DOF, reflecting observations of a subject's classroom behavior. The SCICA was specifically designed to facilitate such comparisons for integrating data from multiple sources. Chapter 8 discusses relations between the SCICA and the CBCL, TRF, and DOF.

SUMMARY

The SCICA provides a flexible semistructured format for interviewing children and adolescents. Structured rating forms are used for scoring the interviewer's observations and the subject's self-reports during the interview. The SCICA

Protocol outlines specific questions and tasks tapping nine broad areas of functioning. Spaces are provided for the interviewer to note observations of the subject's behavior, affect, and interaction style during the interview, along with self-reported problems.

Following the interview, the interviewer scores 120 observation items and 114 self-report items for ages 6-12 or 125 self-report items for ages 13-18. Two open-ended items are provided for adding problems that are not specifically listed on the forms.

For ages 6-12, each item on the SCICA Observation and Self-Report Forms is scored on a 4-point scale. The scores for each item are transferred to syndrome scales displayed on the SCICA Profile for Ages 6-12, which is available in hand-scored and computer-scored versions. The profile consists of five syndrome scales derived from the observation items, three syndrome scales derived from the self-report items, Internalizing and Externalizing scores, and separate total problem scores for the Observation Form and the Self-Report Form.

The profile displays an individual's scale scores in relation to percentiles and normalized T scores derived from a sample of 237 referred subjects aged 6-12. The profile also lists scores for items that are not in the syndrome scales, plus specific items scored only for ages 13-18.

Chapter 3
How to do SCICA Interviews

To administer the SCICA, users must have training and experience in clinical interviewing of children and adolescents. They must also have knowledge of standardized assessment procedures. User qualifications for the SCICA are described on pages iii and iv. Chapter 2 provides specific instructions for administering and scoring the SCICA. Yet, in addition to knowing the administration procedures, users must be prepared to cope with unexpected challenges in interviewing children and adolescents. Young et al. (1987) have outlined several sources of error that can arise from interviews, including the structure or format of questions, characteristics of the respondent, and characteristics of the interviewer. This chapter provides guidelines regarding interview settings, interviewers' appearance, explanations to interviewees, and strategies for facilitating good communication and cooperation during the SCICA. A later section describes our videotape training procedures for the SCICA.

SETTING AND INTERVIEWER APPEARANCE

The SCICA should be conducted in a private, comfortable setting that can ensure confidentiality and facilitate communication. For most cases, only the interviewer and the subject should be present in the room, unless there are specific reasons to include other persons, such as a trainee or an interpreter for a deaf child. The room should have a relaxed, neutral atmosphere, preferably with pictures on the walls and some comfortable furniture. Rooms containing medical instruments, examining tables, and disinfectants are apt to trigger anxieties associated with medical procedures. We recommend that the interviewer and subject sit at a small table to facilitate drawing and note-taking. The interviewer can avoid a test-like format by sitting to the right or left of the subject, rather than on the opposite side of the table. It is also important to provide a comfortable chair appropriate for the subject's size and to allow the subject to leave the table occasionally.

The room should be free of items that could create distractions during the interview. Before interviewing young children, or overactive or aggressive children, it may be necessary to "childproof" the room by clearing desks and tables of papers, pencils, and other loose items that are not needed for the interview. It is especially important to remove potentially risky items, such as letter openers, scissors, and pins, plus tempting gadgets, such as radios, calculators, dictating machines, and electric pencil sharpeners. Personal computers can present a particular problem, since many children expect to play games on them. If a computer cannot be removed, it should be covered. Toys and games that will not be used during the interview should be placed out of sight or in a remote location. It is wise to remove family pictures and personal mementos, since they may deflect attention toward the interviewer and away from the subject's interests and relationships. For adolescents, it is important to avoid "child-like" decor that might undermine their self esteem or willingness to cooperate.

The interviewer's personal appearance can also affect rapport with interviewees. As a general rule, the interviewer should dress in professional attire congruent with community standards and the local environment. A very casual appearance may create the false impression that the interview is to be a play session or an informal conversation. Very casual dress could also undermine the interviewer's "professional authority" for asking sensitive questions. In contrast, a "doctor-like" appearance (e.g., wearing a white coat), could raise fears of medical exams, shots, or invasive procedures. For certain subjects, the gender of the interviewer should be considered, based on referral complaints or other prior knowledge about the subject, or specific research purposes, such as matching the gender of interviewer and interviewee.

EXPLAINING PURPOSE AND CONFIDENTIALITY

The interviewer begins the SCICA by explaining the purpose of the session. It is usually helpful to ask subjects why they think they are being interviewed. This provides opportunities to clarify any misconceptions about the nature of the interview. Young children may have been told that they are going to play games or that they are going to be "tested." Other children may fear that the interview will show they are "crazy" or "stupid," or that the interviewer wants to investigate something they did wrong.

Explanations should be clear and succinct, while conveying essential information. The SCICA Protocol specifies statements for introducing the SCICA and explaining confidentiality. The introductory remarks can be adapted to the subject's cognitive level and to the purposes of the interview. Lengthy introductions should be avoided. Too much adult talk at the beginning of an interview may inhibit subjects from talking about themselves.

Assurances and limits of confidentiality should be clearly stated at the beginning of the SCICA. If the interviewer cannot assure confidentiality (e.g., because certain interview content might be cited in assessment reports), then the introductory remarks should be altered accordingly. If a follow-up meeting is planned with parents or other adults, the subject should be informed of this. To ensure that the subject understands these issues, they can be addressed again at the end of the interview. To do this, the interviewer can briefly summarize key topics that were covered and then ask the subject's permission to discuss relevant issues with other informants, such as parents and teachers. In most cases, the interviewer can protect the confidentiality of the interview by discussing issues in general terms with other informants, rather than by repeating the subject's exact words. Another alternative is to discuss items scored on the CBCL or TRF that reflect key problems raised during the interview.

For most purposes, we recommend audiotaping the SCICA. This reduces reliance on written notes and provides a memory aide for scoring the subject's self-reports. The tape recorder should be placed in view of the subject, but where it will not interfere with the interview. As indicated on the SCICA Protocol, the interviewer can explain use of the recorder by saying, *"We are going to record our talk on this tape recorder to help remember our time together. I will erase the tape after I have finished listening to it."* Tapes should be stored in a safe location and erased after all scoring and written reports are finished.

Some users may choose to videotape the SCICA. Videotaping, of course, limits the locations where the SCICA can be administered. We videotape our research interviews through a one-way mirror. The subject sits at a table facing the mirror. In our pilot research, we found that certain children were distracted or inhibited by knowing they were being videotaped. Therefore, with parental consent and approval of the institutional review board, we did not inform our subjects of the videotaping. For the few subjects who asked about videotaping, we explained the procedures and offered to show them the equipment and a short tape segment after the SCICA was completed. This approach alleviated subjects' concerns and distractions about videotaping during the interview.

In certain circumstances, it may be preferable to inform subjects of videotaping as well as audiotaping. For adolescents, it is usually advisable to disclose all recording procedures, including videotaping. In our interviews with 13-18-year-old subjects, we obtain the subjects' and their parents' permission for videotaping. Videotaping or audiotaping is not recommended when it is likely to reduce a subject's willingness to participate or to discuss sensitive issues.

INTERVIEWING STRATEGIES

Sensitive clinical interviewing requires flexibility in addressing a subject's specific concerns while also focusing on key issues necessary for adequate assessment. As discussed in Chapter 1, children may be unable to respond accurately to highly structured questions about their problems. Adolescents may also resist responding to questions that they perceive as reflecting adult agendas more than their own concerns.

To facilitate communication, the SCICA is designed to be flexible, yet comprehensive in tapping behavioral, social, and emotional functioning. As explained in Chapter 2, the SCICA Protocol outlines topics, questions, and tasks to be covered. Table 3-1 outlines various "do's" and "don'ts" of interviewing strategies, as discussed in the next sections.

Open-Ended Questioning

The open-ended format of most SCICA questions enables interviewers to tailor inquiries to fit subjects' cognitive levels and interaction styles. An example is the question, *"What do you like best in school?"* Common responses are "gym, lunch, and recess." Occasionally, a subject may cite reading, math, or journal writing. Open-ended questions are preferable to questions that can be answered "yes" or "no," because children often reply "yes" or "no" without elaborating. An excess of factual questions may also inhibit subjects because their memory is limited, they are reluctant to disclose information, or they fear being wrong. Questions eliciting feelings, thoughts, or opinions, on the other hand, avoid implying that there are right or wrong answers.

Table 3-1
Interviewing Strategies with the SCICA

_Do's_	_Don'ts_
Use open-ended questions.	Don't make judgmental comments.
Follow the subject's lead in conversation.	Don't use embedded questions and phrases.
Limit the length of questions and comments.	Don't repeat swear words or obscene language.
Ask only one question at a time.	Don't introduce topics and tasks with rhetorical questions, such as "Would you like to ____?"
Rephrase or simplify questions if the subject misunderstands or fails to respond.	
Use the subject's words and terminology.	Avoid asking "why" questions about reasons for behavior.
Use people's names instead of pronouns.	Don't follow every response from the subject with another question.
Use direct requests to introduce certain topics and tasks, such as "Tell me about____."	
Intersperse nonverbal activities with questioning.	

Open-ended requests and questions can be followed by probes for more detailed information. Examples are the questions about peer relationships in Section 2 of the SCICA Protocol: *"Tell me about someone you like. What do you like about _____?"* and *"Tell me about someone you don't like. What don't you like about _____?"* Most subjects will name at least one person they like and one they don't like. The interviewer can then probe further about relations with persons liked and disliked to assess friendships, the nature of contacts with peers, and strategies for coping with peer problems. For example, in answer to the question about someone not liked, a subject may describe a child who hits. The interviewer can then ask, "What do you do when _____ hits you?" or "How does that make you feel when _____ hits you?" This could be followed by asking, "What else could you do when _____ hits you?"

Certain SCICA items begin with a focused question, followed by open-ended questions and requests for the subject's opinion. An example is the series of questions concerning family rules in Section 3 of the SCICA Protocol: *"Who makes the rules in your home? What happens when kids break the rules? Do you think the rules are fair or unfair?"* The next segment in Section 3 begins with an open-ended question about punishments: *"What are the punishments in your home? Who punishes you when you do something wrong? Do you think the punishments are fair or unfair?"* These open-ended questions offer opportunities for describing rules, consequences, and punishments in the home. Some subjects may respond by saying there are no rules or punishments. Others may cite specific rules, such as "no jumping on the furniture," "no fighting," "no swearing," or "no TV until homework is done." Examples of consequences or punishments can include "yelling," "spanking," "being sent to my room," or "being grounded."

If a subject does not spontaneously mention any consequences or punishments, the interviewer can ask more direct questions. Direct questions should initially be phrased in a non-personal way, such as "Do kids get spanked in your home?" or "Do kids get sent to their rooms?" rather than "Do you get spanked?" or "Does you mother send you to your room?" The non-personal questions are likely to elicit more detailed responses than the personally directed questions because they may be less embarrassing and they allow more response options. For example, subjects may report that they get sent to their rooms as punishment, but that younger siblings get spanked. The forced-choice format of the questions regarding fairness (Section 3) also clearly indicates to the subject that either response ("fair" or "unfair") is acceptable. If the interviewer asks only if the rules are fair, this might bias the subject toward a "yes" response. Additional open-ended questions can be used to explore reasons for the subject's views of the fairness or unfairness of family rules and punishments.

Avoiding Judgmental Comments

Judgmental comments can inhibit subjects' spontaneous expression of their thoughts, feelings, and opinions. However, such comments may be difficult to avoid, especially for inexperienced interviewers. This is because adults are accustomed to teaching and controlling children. In response to judgmental comments, children may say what they believe an adult wants to hear or may try to defend themselves from disapproval by saying nothing.

To avoid seeming judgmental, the interviewer can minimize positive and negative reactions to the child's comments or activities. For example, if a boy says that he likes math, do not say, "Oh, that's nice!" or "I bet you're good in math." Instead, it is better to follow up with another open-ended, non-judgmental response, such as "Tell me what you like about math." If a subject says, "I hate math," do not say "Gee that's too bad" or "Math must be hard for you." Instead, the subject's comment can be followed with the question, "What don't you like about math?" If subjects say there is "nothing" they like about school, the interviewer can ask, "Then what do you like least in school?"

For subjects who can't articulate what they like or don't like, more structured probes with a multiple-choice format can be used, such as, "Some kids don't like math because it is hard, or it's boring, or they don't understand it. How do you feel about math?" Multiple-choice probes do not imply approval or disapproval of particular responses. When using structured probes about feelings, it is particularly important to include options that permit the child to say something negative as well as positive about a topic. Even encouraging comments, such as "That sounds like fun," or "I like your drawing," can inhibit children's expression of their own thoughts and feelings, especially if their feelings run counter to the interviewer's comments.

Following the Subject's Lead in Conversation

The SCICA Protocol begins with questions regarding interests and activities to provide a "warm up" prior to discussing more sensitive issues. However, the interviewer is free to address topics that follow the subject's lead in conversation. If the subject digresses from the sequence outlined on the protocol, the interviewer can defer unaddressed topics until later in the interview. In other words, the interviewer can move around the SCICA Protocol in response to cues from the subject. For example, when some children hear the introduction to the SCICA, "I want to learn about what you like and don't like," they immediately respond, "My sister. I don't like my sister!" When such a response occurs, the interviewer can immediately ask some questions about family relations. It is usually preferable, however, to save the family drawing task for later in the interview to provide an alternative to verbal questioning. After the subject's spontaneous comments have been addressed, the interviewer can return to the earlier SCICA topics, such as activities, school, and friends.

Allowing subjects to influence the selection and sequencing of topics helps to keep them interested and talking. However, the meandering, "illogical" nature of young children's conversation can sometimes tempt interviewers to impose more structure. Meandering conversation can also make it hard for interviewers to keep track of what has been discussed if no written protocol is used. The SCICA Protocol is designed to help interviewers keep track of what has been covered. The Protocol should be periodically checked to ensure that all key questions and topics are covered.

Techniques for Promoting Cooperation

Additional "do's" and "don'ts" listed in Table 3-1 are intended to promote cooperation during the SCICA. A key technique is to limit the length of the questions and comments in order to minimize "interviewer talk" and maximize "interviewee talk" as much as possible. Garbarino and Scott (1989) recommend that interviewers limit their questions and comments to three to five more words than the subject's usual sentence length. This may not always be possible or desirable, but is a good "rule of thumb" for monitoring interviewer talk. Asking only one question at a time and avoiding embedded questions and phrases will also reduce interviewer talk, as well as reduce the memory demands on the subject. If subjects misunderstand or fail to respond, the interviewer should simplify the questions.

For young children, incorporating the subjects' own words and terminology into questions can facilitate understanding, especially using their terms for body parts or bodily functions, rules at home and school, and descriptions of activities. The interviewer can ask for these terms explicitly, if necessary. Garbarino and Scott (1989) also suggested using people's names instead of pronouns to avoid confusion in referents. One caveat is not to repeat swear words or obscene language used by subjects. Although this may seem old fashioned, young children, and even adolescents, can easily misinterpret such repetitions as approval. A neutral response to swearing or obscene language is usually sufficient to avoid discouraging subjects' expressions of negative feelings.

Adults often use rhetorical questions as polite commands, such as "Would you like to _____?" However, the intent of such questions can easily be misunderstood by young children. For example, if the interviewer asks, "Would you like to tell me about school?", young children may logically respond "No," especially if they have negative feelings about school. Or if an interviewer asks, "Would you like to draw me a picture of your family doing something together?", a subject may choose not to draw. Young children often interpret such questions as presenting true options for doing or not doing what is requested. Rhetorical questions can also invite noncompliance from older subjects who understand their polite intent, but have oppositional tendencies. As an alternative, an interviewer can make direct requests, such as, "Tell me about school," or "Draw me a picture of your family doing something together. It can be anything you want." Such statements carry a clear message of the interviewer's intent, and can still be said in a friendly and encouraging manner.

Avoiding "why" questions is another way to facilitate cooperation and communication. Adults often ask children "why" questions to solicit reasons for their behavior or their understanding of other people's behavior. However, when children have misbehaved, they may interpret "why" questions as accusations or reprimands. In other cases, children may not know the reasons for their own behavior or the behavior of others. In either situation, "why" questions often produce "I don't know" responses that are difficult to probe further. An alternative is the reflective technique of repeating the subject's responses in follow-up questions and probes. For example, suppose that a girl reports that other children refuse to play with her. Instead of asking "Why won't other kids play with you?", the interviewer might say, "So other kids won't play with you. Tell me more about that. How does that make you feel?" or "What do you do when they won't play with you?"

Interviewers should also avoid following every response from the subject with another question. Instead, the interviewer can make direct requests, such as "Tell me about _____," or can make reflective comments on the subject's response prior to asking a new question, as illustrated in previous examples. Varying the grammatical structure of the interviewer's statements in this way can avoid tedium.

Interspersing Nonverbal Activities with Questioning

Young children and many adolescents may resist direct questioning about their problems. Interspersing nonverbal activities with questioning can help reduce resistance. The Kinetic Family Drawing (KFD) in Section 3 of the SCICA Protocol provides one nonverbal technique for obtaining information about the family. The KFD is used routinely for ages 6-12 and is optional for ages 13-18. After the subject finishes drawing, the interviewer inquires about family members and relationships by asking the questions listed on the Protocol. The interviewer can also inquire about the content of the drawing, such as positioning of family members, persons included or excluded from the drawing, and the subject's fantasies about what might happen next in a story about the drawing.

Play materials can also be used with young children as a nonverbal supplement to questions. Blocks, a doll family, additional adult and child dolls, and doll house furniture can be especially useful. Open-ended questions can be interjected into the child's play to inquire about family relations and activities portrayed in play. However, the SCICA is not a play interview or play therapy technique. Instead, play materials are to be used at the interviewer's discretion to elicit behavior from young children who are difficult to engage in conversation.

The interviewer should inquire about the subject's play or drawing to determine whether they actually reflect problems experienced by the child. For example, if a young child plays violently with doll family figures, the interviewer can comment, "There is a lot of fighting going on in that family. Do people fight like that in your home?" If a child draws a picture of the family with no father or mother, the interviewer can inquire about the missing parent and the subject's feelings toward that parent. These questions help to clarify whether the child's play or drawings depict fantasies or aspects of actual events or circumstances affecting the subject. Such clarifications are needed for scoring of the SCICA Observation and Self-Report Forms. However, the interviewer should rate the observation and self-report items on the basis of actual problems observed or reported during the interview, and not solely on the basis of inferences drawn from play or drawings.

The achievement tests and motor screening in Sections 7 and 8 of the SCICA Protocol provide other alternatives to direct questioning. Although these sections are optional, they offer opportunities to observe subjects' responses to structured school-like tasks and motor activities in contrast to the semistructured interviewing in Sections 1-6. For some subjects, certain problems may become more evident during the structured tasks than during verbal questioning. Other subjects may show marked changes in problems exhibited or reported when they reach the structured sections of the SCICA. For example, certain subjects may show more anxiety and report more school problems during the achievement testing than during open-ended questioning. Other subjects may become more resistant, restless, or manipulative during testing than during interviewing. Still others may become more self-assured and enthusiastic, or start joking and clowning, during testing and motor screening than during earlier portions of the interview. Thus, the achievement tests and motor screening not only provide breaks from verbal questioning, but can also increase the range of potential problems to be observed or reported during the SCICA.

VIDEOTAPE TRAINING PROCEDURES

To provide standardized training in rating SCICA interviews, we offer a videotape showing segments of interviews that have been rated by several experienced raters. The tape can be ordered from the address shown on page ii.

In each segment, a child actor enacts a portion of a real interview with a child who had been referred for mental health services. Child actors and changes in certain details are used to protect the identity of the original subjects.

To use the tape, a trainee should first become fully familiar with the SCICA Observation and Self-Report Forms, as well as with this Manual and the SCICA Protocol. The trainee should then watch an interview segment one or more times, taking extensive notes on what the child does and says. After watching the segment, the trainee scores the Observation and Self-Report Forms on the basis of what has been noted and remembered from the video segment.

Next, the trainee enters the Observation and Self-Report item scores into the SCICA computer scoring program as instructed by the documentation that accompanies the program and videotape. Following the instructions given in the computer program, the trainee then compares the item and scale scores, as well as the profile pattern, obtained from the trainee's own ratings and the mean of the ratings by the experienced raters. Trainees can thus see precisely where their ratings agree and differ from those of experienced raters in terms of item and scale scores, as well as overall profile patterns. The program also prints intraclass correlations (ICCs) between the trainee's scores and those of the experienced raters.

The documentation accompanying the videotape provides guidelines for judging the degree of agreement indicated by the ICCs. If the ICCs are low or there are specific disagreements between ratings by a trainee and the experienced raters, the trainee can watch and rescore the interview segment as many times as necessary to achieve the level of agreement recommended in the documentation accompanying the tape. The videotaped cases encompass a wide range of child characteristics, as illustrated by data on some of these cases in Chapter 10.

SUMMARY

To administer the SCICA, interviewers must have training in clinical interviewing of children, as well as knowledge of standardized assessment. The SCICA should be administered in an appropriate private setting. Confidentiality and its limits are initially explained to the subject.

Effective interviewing strategies include open-ended questioning; avoiding judgmental comments; following the subject's lead in conversation; several techniques for promoting cooperation; and interspersing nonverbal activities with questioning.

To provide standardized training in rating SCICA interviews, a videotape is available that shows segments of interviews. Trainees can watch and score each segment and compare their scores with the mean of scores obtained from experienced raters until they reach good agreement.

Chapter 4
Development of the SCICA
Scoring Forms and Profile

The SCICA was designed to sample children's functioning during a clinical interview, to yield psychometrically sound scores for observed and reported problems, and to provide data that can be meshed with data from other sources. To meet these goals, we employed a psychometric approach for developing the SCICA similar to that used for the CBCL, TRF, YSR, and DOF. This involved constructing standardized rating forms for scoring interviewers' observations and children's self-reports. The data obtained with these forms were then used to derive empirically based scales for the SCICA Profile.

The *Guide for the Semistructured Interview for Children* (McConaughy & Achenbach, 1990) described our initial scoring forms and a provisional profile for ages 6-11. This chapter reports research on an expanded sample to refine the SCICA Observation and Self-Report Forms and to construct the 1994 Profile for Ages 6-12. Chapters 5 and 6 present findings on reliability and validity.

DEVELOPMENT OF THE SCICA
OBSERVATION AND SELF-REPORT FORMS

The items for ages 6-12 on the Observation and Self-Report Forms were assembled from a pool of observation and self-report items as follows:

1. The CBCL was examined to find items appropriate for the interview situation. Whenever possible, the

original wording of the CBCL items was retained. Certain CBCL items were reworded to make them more appropriate for observations during an interview, such as rewording CBCL item *8. Can't concentrate, can't pay attention for long* to SCICA item *31. Doesn't concentrate or pay attention for long on tasks, questions, topics.* Other CBCL items were reworded for rating self-reports of behaviors that were unlikely to be observed in the interview setting. Examples are SCICA items *122. Reports acts of cruelty, bullying or meanness to others, including siblings; 130. Reports being disobedient at home*; and *134. Reports being lonely or left out of others' activities.* The CBCL yielded 50 items for the SCICA Observation Form and 81 items for the SCICA Self-Report Form.

2. The TRF was examined for candidate items beside those that were drawn from the CBCL. Some TRF items were reworded slightly to make them more appropriate for observations or children's self-reports in a fashion similar to the rewording of CBCL items. The TRF yielded 12 items for the Observation Form and 6 items for the Self-Report Form. Examples are *28. Demands must be met immediately*; *29. Difficulty following directions*; and *159. Reports disliking school or work.*

3. Additional items were developed from reviews of the literature, our own observations during clinical work and pilot research on the SCICA, and comments that were added on the open-ended items during initial phases of data collection. Examples include: *3. Giggles too much; 9. Avoids eye contact; 30. Disjointed or tangential conversation; 40. Frequently off task; 61. Misbehaves, taunts, or tests the limits; 76. Resistant or refuses to comply (describe); 135. Reports being physically harmed by parent or guardian*

(describe); 136. Reports being punished a lot at home, including spanking (describe); 150. Reports concerns about family problems (describe); and *215. Talks about death, including deaths of animals, family members, etc. (describe).* This yielded 62 items for the Observation Form and 39 items for the Self-Report Form.

4. Using the item scores for the 1990 sample of 108 subjects, we computed frequencies and correlations among items for both SCICA forms separately. Six observation items were then eliminated because they were never scored as present by either the interviewer or the observer. Two highly correlated observation items were combined. Eighteen self-report items were eliminated because they were never scored, and two were combined into one item because they covered very similar topics. Certain items with low frequencies were retained in view of their clinical significance, such as *11. Behaves like opposite sex; 154. Reports deliberately harming self or attempting suicide; 195. Reports running away from home;* and *198. Reports setting fires.* This resulted in a reduction of the item pool to 117 items for the 1990 version of the Observation Form and 107 items for the 1990 Self-Report Form, plus an open-ended item for reporting additional problems on each form.

5. As our research on the SCICA advanced, we developed three new items for the 1994 Observation Form: *118. Denies responsibility or blames others*; *119. Flat affect*; and *120. Overly dramatic.* We developed seven new items for the 1994 Self-Report Form: *220. Talks about getting revenge without physical attack; 221. Reports being mad or angry; 222. Reports strange behavior; 223. Reports conflict with family re: plans for work or education; 224. Reports conflict with family re: social activities;*

225. Reports problems in sexual identity or concern about homosexuality; and *226. Reports problems in social relations with opposite sex.* Items were also renumbered to accommodate the additional items and to group somatic complaints together (items 228-235) at the end of page 4 on the Self-Report Form. For ages 6-12, there are 120 items on the 1994 SCICA Observation Form and 114 items on the 1994 Self-Report Form, plus an open-ended item for additional problems on each form.

6. In addition to the 1994 Observation and Self-Report items for ages 6-12, we developed items for scoring self-reports for ages 13-18. These include items 228-235, which cover the same somatic complaints scored for ages 6-12, but use different anchor points for scores of *1, 2,* and *3.* Eleven new items were added (items 236-246) to cover problems specific to ages 13-18. However, none of the items specific to ages 13-18 were included in the statistical derivation of the syndrome scales for ages 6-12.

SAMPLE FOR DEVELOPING THE SCICA

The research sample for developing the 1990 provisional profile consisted of 108 6- to 11-year-old children referred for evaluation of behavioral/emotional or learning problems. To develop the 1994 Profile for Ages 6-12, the original sample was expanded to 168 referred subjects aged 6-12. Subjects were referred to the Center for Children, Youth, and Families at the University of Vermont Department of Psychiatry or for psychoeducational assessments in their schools. To avoid the possible effects of low cognitive ability or physical problems on behavior, children were excluded if they had a full scale IQ below 75 or physical disabilities or disorders, such as epilepsy. Parents were asked for permission to interview the child as part of a research study on interviews. Parents were offered the option of subsequently meeting with the interviewer to discuss the clinical impressions and achievement test results obtained during the interview. Subjects were paid for their participation in the research.

As part of the evaluation, at least one parent of each subject completed the CBCL and a background information form. With parental permission, the TRF was obtained from teachers. An independent observer used the DOF to score 75 subjects who were observed on three occasions in their classrooms.

The final sample included 119 boys and 49 girls, with a mean age of 8.7 years (*s.d.* = 1.8). With one exception, the subjects were caucasian. Parental socioeconomic status (SES) was scored according to Hollingshead's (1975) 9-step scale for occupation, where 9 = highest SES. If both parents were wage earners, the higher status occupation was used. The mean SES was 5.4 (*s.d.* = 2.3). Table 4-1 lists the ages and SES.

INTERVIEWING AND
SCORING PROCEDURES

Subjects were interviewed by Dr. McConaughy or two other psychologists at the Center for Children, Youth, and Families. Each interview was videotaped through a one-way mirror. Parents granted informed consent for their children to be videotaped. Most interviews were also audiotaped on a recorder that was shown to the child. The interviewer explained the procedure to the subject according to the standard instructions on the SCICA Protocol by saying: "*We are going to spend some time talking and doing things together, so that I can get to know you and learn about what you like and don't like. This is a private talk. I won't tell your parents or your teachers what you say unless you tell me it is OK. The only thing I might tell is if you said you were going to hurt yourself, hurt someone else, or someone*

Table 4-1
Age and Socioeconomic Status of Referred Sample
Used to Derive SCICA Scales

	Boys N = 119	Girls N = 49	Combined N = 168
Age	% (N)	% (N)	% (N)
6	13 (15)	8 (4)	11 (19)
7	19 (22)	22 (11)	19 (33)
8	16 (19)	22 (11)	18 (30)
9	20 (24)	20 (10)	20 (34)
10	13 (15)	8 (4)	11 (19)
11	13 (15)	12 (6)	13 (21)
12	8 (9)	6 (3)	7 (12)
Mean	8.7	8.6	8.7
S.D.	1.8	1.7	1.8
SES[a]			
Upper	34 (40)	47 (23)	38 (63)
Middle	40 (48)	35 (17)	39 (65)
Lower	26 (31)	18 (9)	24 (40)
Mean	5.3	5.7	5.4
S.D.	2.2	2.3	2.3

Note. Because of rounding, columns may not sum to 100%.
[a]Hollingshead (1975) 9-step scale for parental occupation, using the higher status occupation if both parents were wage earners; scores 1-3.5 = Lower; 4-6.5 = Middle; 7-9 = Upper.

has hurt you. We are going to record our talk on this tape recorder to help remember our time together."

In 94 of the 168 cases (56%), the interviewer was kept blind to the referral complaints.   In other cases, the interviewer was familiar with the subject's background prior to the evaluation. However, for all subjects, the interviewer was kept blind to the six parent- or teacher-reported problems that were listed in Section 6 of the SCICA Protocol prior to addressing them in the interview. The six problems were entered on the Protocol by an assistant who selected them from items scored 2 (*very true or often true*) by parents on the CBCL or by teachers on the TRF. In the few cases where fewer than six CBCL or TRF items were scored 2, the assistant added problems scored *1* or problems reported as specific referral concerns.

After the SCICA was completed, the interviewer scored the subject on each item of the Observation and Self-Report Forms. A rater who was blind as to the subject's background and presenting problems also viewed the videotaped interview and scored the subject on the SCICA rating forms. Ratings obtained from the interviewer and a videotape observer were averaged to increase the reliability of each subject's scores for analysis. Across the sample of 168 subjects, ratings were provided by a total of three interviewers and seven videotape observers.

STATISTICAL DERIVATION OF SYNDROMES FOR AGES 6-12

To develop the 1994 syndrome scales for ages 6-12, we performed statistical analyses modeled on those used to develop the syndrome scales for the CBCL, TRF, and YSR. We did this by performing separate principal components analyses of the observation and self-report items for the sample of 168 referred subjects. Like factor analysis, principal components analysis is used to identify groups of items whose scores covary with each other. In factor analysis, the obtained correlations among items are reduced to reflect only the variance each item has in common with all other items (*communality*). An item's communality is typically estimated by the squared multiple correlation between the item and all other items. In principal components analysis, the obtained correlations among items are taken at face value rather than being reduced by communality estimates. To accomplish this, principal components analysis uses 1.0 in the principal diagonal of the correlation matrix instead of communality estimates for individual items. When the number of items is large, the results of principal components analysis are generally similar to those of factor analysis (Gorsuch, 1983).

Before performing the principal components analyses, we tabulated the frequency of each item to identify items that were too rarely endorsed to contribute meaningfully to the analyses. We excluded items that were endorsed by either the interviewer or the videotape observer for less than 5% of the 168 subjects. This resulted in 111 items from the Observation Form and 81 items from the Self-Report Form that were submitted to separate principal components analyses. Table 4-2 lists the items excluded from the principal components analyses.

To determine which problems occurred together to form syndromes, we computed Pearson correlations among the 111 observation items and among the 81 self-report items, using the mean of the interviewer's and videotape observer's ratings of each item for each subject. After performing principal components analyses, we subjected the largest 3 to 9 components from each analysis to orthogonal (varimax) rotations in order to identify syndromes that remained relatively intact despite changes in the number of components. (Rotations of principal components are transformations of their item loadings to approximate the ideal of "simple structure," that is, to divide all items analyzed into relatively tightly knit groups of strongly interrelated items.)

Table 4-2
Low Frequency Items Excluded from
Principal Components Analyses

Observation Items	*Self-Report Items*	
11. Behaves like opposite sex	125. Rpts behaving like opposite sex	211. Rpts wetting bed
13. Bizarre language	129. Rpts cruelty to animals	212. Rpts daytime wetting
37. Feels guilty	146. Rpts being underactive	213. Rpts wishing to be opposite sex
47. Hears things	148. Rpts BM outside toilet	216. Talks about harming self
90. Stares at interviewer	149. Rpts compulsive acts	217. Rpts sexual problems
118. Denies responsibility	154. Rpts harming self	220. Talks about revenge
119. Flat affect	163. Rpts fearing school	221. Rpts being angry
120. Overly dramatic	166. Rpts feeling hurt when criticized	222. Rpts strange behavior
	180. Rpts hearing things	223. Rpts conflict w. family re: education
	184. Rpts neglect	224. Rpts conflict w. family re: social activities
	195. Rpts running away	225. Rpts problems in sexual identity
	198. Rpts setting fires	226. Rpts problems with opposite sex
	202. Rpts storing up things	227. Rpts alcohol/ drug use
	206. Rpts thinking about sex	230. Rpts nausea
	209. Rpts truancy	231. Rpts overeating
	210. Rpts vandalism	233. Rpts rashes
		235. Rpts vomiting

The 5-component rotation for the Observation Form and the 4-component rotation for the Self-Report Form produced the most robust syndromes. We retained components comprising ≥10 items with loadings ≥.30 as the basis for constructing the syndrome scales of the SCICA Profile. Applying these criteria, we retained all five components from the 5-component rotation of the observation items, and three components from the 4-component rotation of the self-report items. Eigenvalues (the sum of squared loadings of all items) of the retained rotated components ranged from 4.69 to 12.61 for the Observation Form and from 3.84 to 5.80 for the Self-Report Form.

To select final item sets for the SCICA syndrome scales, we considered all items that loaded ≥.30 on one or more components. From the 5-component rotation of the observation items, four items loaded highest on the first component and ≥.30 on one or more of the remaining four components. Because of the large proportion of variance accounted for by the first component (eigenvalue = 12.61), we followed the procedure used with the large first component of the CBCL, TRF, and YSR, whereby we assigned these four cross-loading items to the component on which they had their second highest loading. All items loading ≥.30 on the first component of the 4-component rotation of the self-report items were retained on that component since they did not load ≥.30 on any other component. All other observation and self-report items that loaded ≥.30 on more than one component were retained on the component on which they had their highest loading.

We selected names for the syndrome scales that summarized the content of each scale. Four syndromes were similar enough to the CBCL, TRF, and YSR cross-informant syndromes to warrant similar names, while four other syndromes were more unique to the SCICA. The five syndromes derived from the Observation Form were designated as *Anxious*,[OB] *Attention Problems*,[OB] *Resistant*,[OB] *Strange*,[OB] and *Withdrawn*.[OB] The three syndromes derived from the Self-Report Form were designated as *Anxious/ Depressed*,[SR] *Family Problems*,[SR] and *Aggressive Behavior*.[SR] (The superscripts *OB* and *SR* indicate the forms from which the syndromes were derived.) Appendix B lists the items according to their loadings on the eight syndrome scales.

INTERNALIZING AND EXTERNALIZING GROUPINGS OF SYNDROMES

Because broad groupings of problems may also be useful for judging a child's functioning, we performed second-order principal factor analyses of the raw scores obtained by the 168 subjects on the syndrome scales. Principal factor analyses were used instead of principal components analyses because factor analysis has been shown to be superior in applications to small numbers of variables, such as our eight syndrome scales (Snook & Gorsuch, 1989). As a first step, we computed total raw scores for each of the eight syndrome scales by summing the mean of the interviewer's and observer's ratings (*0, 1, 2, 3*) for all items of a scale for each subject. We then computed Pearson correlations among subjects' total scores on each of the eight syndromes. We performed principal factor analyses of the correlations among the syndromes, followed by orthogonal (varimax) rotations of 2 and 3 factors. The 2-factor solution contained factors that corresponded to the dichotomy between Internalizing and Externalizing problems identified for the CBCL, TRF, and YSR, and in other research.

The Resistant, Strange, Attention Problems, and Aggressive Behavior syndromes had loadings from .42 to .56 on the first factor, which was labeled Externalizing. The Anxious and Anxious/Depressed syndromes had loadings of .55 and .62, respectively, on the second factor, which was labeled Internalizing. The Family Problems syndrome loaded .31 on the Internalizing factor, but this was deemed too weak to warrant including it in the Internalizing grouping of syndromes. The Withdrawn syndrome did not load ≥.30

on either the Internalizing or Externalizing factor. Table 4-3 lists the SCICA syndrome scales in terms of the Internalizing and Externalizing groupings. Eigenvalues for each syndrome obtained from the initial principal components analyses are shown in parentheses.

Table 4-3
Syndromes Derived from Principal
Components/Varimax Analyses

Internalizing	Neither Internalizing nor Externalizing		Externalizing	
Anxious/ Depressed^{SR} (5.53)	Family Problems^{SR}	(3.84)	Aggressive Behavior^{SR}	(5.80)
Anxious^{OB} (5.45)	Withdrawn^{OB}	(10.43)	Attention Problems^{OB}	(4.69)
			Strange^{OB}	(4.91)
			Resistant^{OB}	(12.61)

Note. Syndromes are listed from top left to bottom right according to their loadings on the Internalizing and Externalizing factors. The numbers in parentheses are eigenvalues for each syndrome in principal components/varimax analyses. OB = Observation syndromes; SR = Self-Report syndromes.

ASSIGNING NORMALIZED T SCORES TO RAW SCORES

To assign standard scores to raw scores, we computed the cumulative frequency distribution of total scores obtained on each SCICA scale for a sample of 237 referred children. Scores from the 165 boys and 72 girls were weighted equally. The sample included the 168 subjects used for the statistical derivation of the SCICA scales, plus 69 additional children aged 6-12 who were referred for mental health or special education services. The sample of 237 subjects had a mean age of 8.7 (*s.d.* = 1.6) and mean SES of 5.4 (*s.d.* =

2.2). For the 168 subjects on whom we had interviewer and observer ratings, we used the mean of these ratings for each item. However, because interviews with the remaining 69 subjects were not videotaped, only interviewer ratings were used for these subjects. We assigned normalized T scores to raw scores as described below.

T Scores for the SCICA Syndromes

We computed the cumulative frequency distribution of the total raw scores for each of the eight SCICA syndrome scales. We then assigned normalized T scores to raw scores at each percentile for scores falling between approximately the 11th and 93rd percentiles. The percentiles indicated on the 1994 profile were derived according to a procedure designed to produce smoother, more normal distributions of percentile scores than were generated for the 1990 version of the profile. According to this procedure, a raw score that falls at a particular percentile of the cumulative frequency distribution is assumed to span all the next lower percentiles down to the percentile occupied by the next lower raw score in the distribution (Crocker & Algina, 1986). To represent this span of percentiles, each raw score is assigned to the midpoint of the percentiles that it spans.

As an example, 24.4% of the sample obtained a raw score of 5 or lower on the Anxious/Depressed syndrome. The next higher raw score, 6, was obtained by 4.9% of the subjects. The *cumulative percent* of children obtaining a raw score of 5 or lower was thus 24.4%, while the cumulative percent obtaining a raw score of 6 or lower was 24.4% + 4.9% = 29.3%. The interval from raw score 5 to raw score 6 thus spanned from a cumulative percent of 24.4% to a cumulative percent of 29.3%. To represent this interval in terms of a percentile at the midpoint of the interval, we took the cumulative percent at the top of the interval (29.3%) and subtracted the cumulative percent at the bottom of the interval (24.4%), i.e., 29.3% minus 24.4% = 4.9%. To obtain the midpoint, we then divided this difference in half and added it to the lower percent, i.e., 24.4% + 2.5% = 26.9%. This corresponds to the following formula provided by Crocker and Algina (1986, p. 439):

$$P = \frac{cf_l + .5(f_i)}{N} \ X \ 100\%$$

where P = percentile; cf_l is the cumulative frequency for all scores lower than the score of interest; f_i is the frequency of scores in the interval of interest; and N is the number in the sample.

After obtaining the midpoint percentile in this way, we used the procedure provided by Abramowitz and Stegun (1968) to assign a normalized T score of 44 to the 26.9th percentile for the raw score of 6. The main effect of using the midpoint percentile rather than the cumulative percentile on the syndrome scales was to provide a smoother, less skewed, and more differentiated basis for T scores.

For extremely high and low scores, we departed from basing T scores on percentiles in the following ways:

1. Low scores. We assigned a T score of 38 to all raw scores that fell at about the 11th percentile or below. This procedure equalized the starting points of the scales and is intended to prevent overinterpretation of minor differences at the low end of the scale. All raw scores with a T score of 38 are grouped at the bottom of the SCICA Profile for Ages 6-12.

2. High scores. Most scores above about the 93rd percentile were outliers. For scale scores above the 93rd percentile ($T = 65$), we therefore assigned raw scores to T scores in equal intervals from 66 to 100.

T Scores for Internalizing and Externalizing

We constructed Internalizing and Externalizing groupings from the items that comprised the SCICA syndromes loading ≥.42 on the Internalizing and Externalizing factors in the second-order analyses. We then computed the cumulative frequency distributions of total raw scores for Internalizing and Externalizing. These distributions were used to assign normalized *T* scores to raw scores at each percentile up to the 93rd percentile. We assigned *T* scores to the extremes of the distributions in the following ways:

1. **Low scores**. We assigned a *T* score of 25 to all possible scores up to and including the lowest score actually obtained in our sample of 237 subjects.

2. **High scores**. For Internalizing, we assigned *T* scores of 66 to 100 in equal intervals to all possible raw scores above the 93rd percentile (raw scores 33 to 102). Because the Externalizing scale had so many raw scores above $T = 65$, we assigned 3 raw scores to each *T* score from 66 to 99 (raw scores 56 to 157). We assigned all remaining possible raw scores to a *T* score of 100 because these high scores (ranging up to 219) are likely to be so rare that it is unnecessary to differentiate among them.

T Scores for Total Problem Scores

Total problem scores were obtained for the Observation Form by summing ratings for items 1-120, plus the highest score for any problems added on the open-ended item 121. Total problem scores for the Self-Report Form were obtained by summing ratings for items 122-235, plus the highest score for any problems added on the open-ended item 247. We assigned normalized *T* scores to the total raw scores at each midpoint percentile of the cumulative frequency distribution

up to the 93rd percentile ($T = 65$). T scores were assigned
to the extremes of the distributions in the following ways:

1. **Low scores**. We assigned a T score of 25 to all total
    raw scores up to and including the lowest score
    actually found in our sample of 237 subjects.

2. **High scores**. Because there were so many possible
    scores above the 93rd percentile (ranging up to 363
    on the Observation Form and 345 on the Self-Report
    Form), we assigned 3 raw scores to each T score
    from 66 to 99. We then assigned all the remaining
    possible raw scores to $T = 100$. As with External-
    izing, the raw total scores that receive $T = 100$ are
    unlikely to occur. However, if maximal differentia-
    tion is desired for statistical purposes, raw total
    scores can be used instead of T scores.

SUMMARY

The 1994 SCICA scoring forms and profile were
developed on 168 6- to 12-year-olds who had been referred
for mental health or special education services. Subjects
were interviewed according to the SCICA Protocol and rated
by the interviewer on the SCICA Observation and Self-
Report Forms. Each interview was also videotaped and rated
by an observer of the videotape. Scores from the interviewers and videotape observers were used in statistical analyses
to refine the SCICA rating form and to develop empirically
based scales for ages 6-12.

Items for the Observation and Self-Report Forms were
selected from the CBCL and TRF, plus items developed
specifically for the SCICA. The item pool was reduced to
120 observation items and 114 self-report items by
eliminating those that were rarely scored as present and
combining redundant items. Two open-ended items are also

included for scoring observations and self-reports not covered by specific items.

The SCICA syndrome scales were developed by performing principal components analyses separately for 111 observation items and 81 self-report items scored by the interviewer or videotape observer for at least 5% of the 168 subjects. To increase the reliability of item scores, the interviewer and observer ratings were averaged for use in principal components analyses. The five syndromes derived from the observation items were designated as *Anxious*, *Attention Problems*, *Resistant*, *Strange*, and *Withdrawn*. The three syndromes derived from the self-report items were designated as *Anxious/Depressed*, *Family Problems*, and *Aggressive Behavior*. Second-order principal factor analyses yielded broad Internalizing and Externalizing groupings of these syndromes. The Internalizing grouping included the Anxious and Anxious/Depressed syndromes, while the Externalizing grouping included the Aggressive Behavior, Attention Problems, Resistant, and Strange syndromes.

Normalized *T* scores were assigned to the eight syndrome scales, Internalizing, Externalizing, and the total scores of the Observation Form and the Self-Report Form. The SCICA Profile for Ages 6-12 displays the distributions of raw scores and *T* scores for all scales, as well as percentiles for the eight syndromes, based on 237 referred children.

Chapter 5
Reliability

Reliability refers to agreement between repeated assessments when the phenomena being assessed are expected to remain constant. Because the SCICA is designed to obtain interviewers' and observers' ratings of children's functioning during a clinical interview, it is important to know the degree to which two different raters obtain similar results, i.e., the degree of *inter-rater reliability*. It is also important to know the degree to which raters provide the same scores over periods when the subjects' behavior and self-reports are not expected to change, i.e., *test-retest reliability*. This chapter presents inter-rater reliability between interviewers and videotape observers for 168 subjects and test-retest reliabilities for 20 subjects interviewed twice at intervals averaging 12 days. Because Time 1 and Time 2 interviews were conducted by two different interviewers, *inter-interviewer reliabilities* are also provided as a measure of the degree to which different interviewers obtained similar results. As an additional measure of reliability, *internal consistencies* are listed in Appendix C for each SCICA scale. These are correlations between half of a scale's items and the other half of its items.

Our main purpose in designing the SCICA was to develop empirically based interview procedures. However, we were also interested in determining how the SCICA results related to categorical psychiatric diagnoses, since this has been a major focus of other structured and semistructured child interviews. Inter-rater reliabilities are provided for DSM-III diagnoses made by interviewers and videotape observers, based on the SCICA, CBCL, TRF, and the subjects' clinic records.

INTER-RATER RELIABILITY

To assess inter-rater reliability, interviews were video-taped for 168 referred subjects, as explained in Chapter 4. Interviewers and videotape observers rated each subject on the SCICA Observation and Self-Report Forms. For 56% of the subjects, interviewers were blind to the referral complaints. Observers were blind to referral complaints for all subjects. Ratings were obtained from three interviewers and seven videotape observers. We analyzed agreement between interviewers and videotape observers in two ways: *(1)* Pearson correlations, symbolized by *r*, which mainly reflect similarities in the *rank ordering* between two sets of scores; and *(2)* *t* tests, which reflect differences between the *mean magnitudes* of two sets of scores. The first column of Table 5-1 displays the Pearson *r*s between the interviewer and observer ratings for raw scores on each SCICA scale.

All correlations were significant at *p* <.001, with *r*s ranging from .45 to .80. Reliabilities were highest (*r* >.70) for Family Problems, Withdrawn, Aggressive Behavior, Resistant, and Externalizing, and lowest for Anxious. Means and standard deviations for interviewer and observer ratings are listed in the second and third columns of Table 5-1. Dependent *t* tests showed that mean scores from interviewers were higher than mean scores from observers on all SCICA scales, *p* <.01. Additional *t* tests showed that, averaged across all scales, interviewers scored more items than did observers, *p* <.001, and they tended to assign higher scores to items (more *2*s and *3*s) than did observers, *p* <.001. Interviewing subjects thus appears to lead to more awareness of problems than does viewing videotaped interviews.

Table 5-1
Inter-Rater Reliabilities, Means, and Standard Deviations
for Interviewer and Observer Ratings on SCICA Scales

Scale	Interviewer-Observer r^a	Interviewer Mean^b	S.D.	Observer Mean	S.D.
Anxious/Depressed^{SR}	.69	10.5	7.1	8.2	6.7
Anxious^{OB}	.45	6.1	5.9	2.4	2.9
Family Problems^{SR}	.76	3.2	3.7	2.3	3.4
Withdrawn^{OB}	.76	9.6	10.9	8.1	10.0
Aggressive Behavior^{SR}	.76	6.1	5.8	5.2	5.5
Attention Problems^{OB}	.57	9.9	5.9	7.6	6.2
Strange^{OB}	.69	5.4	5.7	3.9	4.6
Resistant^{OB}	.80	9.0	9.7	7.3	10.1
Internalizing	.64	16.5	11.2	10.5	8.1
Externalizing	.72	30.3	18.1	24.0	18.6
Total Observations	.52	46.2	20.9	33.4	21.2
Total Self-Reports	.58	32.1	14.8	25.1	14.6

Note. Correlations are Pearson *r*s between raw scores obtained from interviewers and videotape observers for 168 referred children aged 6-12. OB = Observation Form; SR = Self-Report Form.
^{a} All *r*s were significant at $p < .001$.
^{b} Interviewer > Observer for all scales, $p < .001$.

TEST-RETEST AND INTER-INTERVIEWER RELIABILITY

To assess test-retest reliability, the SCICA was administered to 20 referred subjects seen by different interviewers over intervals ranging from 7 to 22 days (mean = 12 days). The test-retest sample included 15 boys and 5 girls aged 6-12 (mean age = 8.3; *s.d.* = 1.7). The mean SES of the sample was 5.8 (*s.d.*) = 2.5). One of the test-retest SCICAs was administered to all 20 subjects by the same person, while the other SCICA was administered by one of two other interviewers in counterbalanced order. The counterbalancing of interviewers avoided confounding interviewer effects with Time 1 versus Time 2 order effects. The test-retest reliabilities obtained in this way provide an especially rigorous test of consistency over time despite three sources of variance: different interviewers administering the SCICA, different raters (interviewers) scoring the SCICA, and changes in subjects' behavior from Time 1 to Time 2.

Pearson rs were used to assess agreement between Time 1 and Time 2 interviews and between interviewers. Time and interviewer effects on mean scores were tested with 2 x 2 ANOVAs, as explained later. Because Pearson r reflects similarities between the rank orders of scores obtained at Time 1 and Time 2, it is high when ratings of individual subjects retain approximately the same rank from Time 1 to Time 2. Because it is not affected by the absolute magnitude of scores, r can be high even if all the Time 1 scores differ in magnitude from the Time 2 scores. ANOVAs, by contrast, test the differences between mean scores relative to their variance. A main effect of Time could, therefore, indicate that there was a significant difference between Time 1 and Time 2 mean scores, even if individuals did not change their ranks from Time 1 to Time 2. By reporting both the rs and the ANOVA results, we enable users to consider test-retest consistency separately in terms of the rank order and magnitude of scores.

The first column of Table 5-2 shows test-retest rs between scores for Time 1 versus Time 2. The test-retest rs were significant ($p \leq .01$) for all scales except Withdrawn. Test-retest reliabilities were highest ($r \geq .70$) for Anxious, Attention Problems, Strange, Resistant, Externalizing, total Observation score, and total Self-Report score. These results indicated good test-retest reliability for most SCICA scales.

The second column of Table 5-2 shows the rs between scores obtained by the interviewer who saw all the subjects and the other interviewers. Like the test-retest rs, the inter-interviewer rs were significant ($p < .01$) for all scales except

Table 5-2
Test-Retest and Inter-Interviewer Reliabilities of SCICA Scales

Scale	Test-Retest r	Inter-Interviewer r
Anxious/Depressed[SR]	.54	.66
Anxious[OB]	.75	.78
Family Problems[SR]	.60	.60
Withdrawn[OB]	(.30)	(.34)
Aggressive Behavior[SR]	.67	.68
Attention Problems[OB]	.71	.82
Strange[OB]	.72	.68
Resistant[OB]	.74	.74
Internalizing	.69	.72
Externalizing	.84	.85
Total Observations	.89	.90
Total Self-Reports	.73	.75

Note. Correlations are Pearson *r*s for raw scores obtained from two different interviewers for 20 children over a mean interval of 12 days. The first column shows *r*s between Time 1 and Time 2, while the second column shows *r*s between different interviewers. All *r*s were significant at $p \leq .01$, except the ones in parentheses. OB = Observation Form; SR = Self-Report Form.

Withdrawn. Inter-interviewer reliabilities were highest ($r > .70$) for Anxious, Attention Problems, Resistant, Internalizing, Externalizing, total Observation score, and total Self-Report score.

Time and interviewer effects on mean scores were tested in two sets of 2 x 2 ANOVAs. One set of ANOVAs employed a 2 (Time 1 vs. Time 2 repeated measures) x 2 (interviewer sequence) design. ("Interviewer sequence" refers to whether the person who interviewed all subjects conducted the first or second interview.) These ANOVAs tested the difference between Time 1 versus Time 2 scores across the two interviewer sequences, separately for each scale. No significant differences were found between Time 1 and Time 2 scores nor between the two interviewer sequences on any scale. Although the sample was relatively small, the SCICA thus did not manifest the tendency for problem scores to decline markedly from the first to the second interview (attenuation effect) that has been found in the DISC (Edelbrock et al., 1985; Jensen et al., 1994).

The closest to a significant difference between Time 1 and Time 2 scores was on the observation items of the Strange scale, where the p value reached .17. The total Self-Report score, which provided the strongest test of an attenuation effect on self-reported problems, yielded an F value of 0.09, $p = .76$, indicating virtually no difference between problems reported by subjects at Time 1 versus Time 2. There were significant interactions between Time 1 versus Time 2 scores and interviewer sequence on two scales, which is no more than expected by chance (Sakoda et al., 1954).

The second set of 2 x 2 ANOVAs tested the difference between scores obtained by the interviewer who interviewed all subjects versus the other two interviewers across interviewer sequence, separately for each scale. These ANOVAs showed significant interviewer differences on two scales, which is no more than expected by chance (Sakoda et al., 1954). There were no significant effects of interviewer sequence nor interactions between interviewer and sequence.

INTERNAL CONSISTENCY

A property of scales that is sometimes referred to as "reliability" is their internal consistency. This is the correlation between half of a scale's items and the other half of its items. Although internal consistency is called "split-half reliability," it cannot tell us the degree to which a scale will produce the same results over different occasions when the target phenomena are expected to remain constant. Furthermore, some scales with relatively low internal consistency may be more *valid* than some scales with very high internal consistency. For example, if a scale consists of 25 repetitions of exactly the same item, it should produce very high internal consistency, because respondents should repeatedly score the same item in the same way on a particular occasion. However, such a scale may be less valid than a scale that uses 25 different items to assess the same phenomenon. If each of the 25 different items taps different aspects of the target phenomenon and is subject to different errors of measurement, the 25 different items are likely to provide better measurement despite lower internal consistency than a scale that repeats the same item 25 times.

The SCICA syndrome scales were derived from principal components analyses of the correlations among items. The composition of the syndrome scales is therefore based on correlations among certain subsets of items. Measures of the internal consistency of the syndrome scales are thus somewhat redundant with the inter-item correlations on which the scales were based. Nevertheless, because some users may wish to know the internal consistency of the SCICA scales, Cronbach's (1951) *alpha* was computed for each scale using a demographically matched sample of 53 referred and 53 nonreferred subjects ($N = 106$). (Details of the sample and matching procedures are described in Chapter 6.) *Alpha* represents the mean of the correlations between all possible sets of half the items comprising a scale. The *alpha* coefficients ranged from .81 to .86 and are displayed in Appendix C for the eight SCICA syndromes, Internalizing, Externalizing, total Observation score, and total Self-Report score.

AGREEMENT ON DSM DIAGNOSES

After rating a subject on the SCICA Observation and Self-Report Forms, the interviewer and videotape observer each assigned a DSM-III diagnosis (American Psychiatric

Association, 1980) based on the SCICA, CBCL, TRF, and information in the child's clinic record. DSM-III diagnoses were obtained in this way for 106 referred children. (DSM-III was used because it was the prevailing nosology when we began our research on the SCICA in 1984.)

Both raters assigned at least one DSM-III diagnosis to 95 of the 106 children. We divided the diagnoses into 13 broad diagnostic categories. A child with multiple diagnoses could be included in more than one diagnostic category. We then computed kappa coefficients (a measure of agreement for categorical data) to determine the level of agreement between the two raters. Table 5-3 lists kappas for the seven diagnostic categories that were used for >3 subjects by both raters.

Table 5-3
DSM-III Diagnoses Based on
SCICA, CBCL, TRF, and Clinic Record

Diagnostic Categories	Number of Diagnoses Interviewer	Observer	Agreement Kappa
Attention Deficit Disorder	41	28	.51
Conduct Disorder	23	19	.70
Oppositional Disorder	9	9	.76
Anxiety Disorder	14	11	.77
Depressive Disorder	16	21	.71
Adjustment Disorder with Mixed Emotions & Conduct	22	9	.45
Learning Disability	21	12	.33

Note. $N = 106$. Table includes diagnostic categories used for >3 subjects by both raters. Subjects with multiple diagnoses are counted for each diagnosis. All kappas were significant at $p < .01$.

As indicated in Table 5-3, the subjects received a variety of diagnoses. Relatively high agreement (kappa $\geq .70$) was found for conduct disorder, oppositional disorder, anxiety disorder, and depressive disorder. There was moderate agreement on attention deficit disorder (kappa = .51), and lower agreement on adjustment disorder and learning disability (kappa ≤.45). The kappas thus indicate satisfactory agreement on five major diagnostic categories when SCICA results were combined with information from other sources.

SUMMARY

Inter-rater reliabilities between SCICA interviewers and observers of videotaped interviews were all significant at p <.001. They ranged from .45 to .80, with 5 of the 12 exceeding .70. Interviewers' ratings were significantly higher than observers' ratings on all scales.

To assess test-retest reliability, the SCICA was administered twice in counterbalanced order by different interviewers at intervals averaging 12 days. Test-retest reliabilities ranged from .54 to .89 (p ≤.01) on all scales except Withdrawn, where the r of .30 was not significant. Inter-interviewer reliabilities on the same sample ranged from .60 to .90 (p <.01) on all scales except Withdrawn, where the r of .34 was not significant. No differences between scores obtained at Time 1 versus Time 2 approached significance on any SCICA scale. Interviewer differences and effects of interviewer sequence did not exceed chance expectations.

Internal consistencies for the SCICA scales ranged from .81 to .86. Kappa coefficients showed moderate to high agreement between interviewers and videotape observers for five categories of DSM-III diagnoses based on the SCICA, parent and teacher ratings, and clinic records.

Chapter 6
Validity

Validity concerns the accuracy with which a procedure measures what it is supposed to measure. The SCICA is designed to measure children's observed and self-reported problems during a semistructured clinical interview. Data obtained from the SCICA are intended to be meshed with data from other sources, particularly the CBCL and TRF. Like other procedures for assessing behavioral/emotional problems, the validity of the SCICA must be evaluated in relation to a variety of criteria, none of which is definitive by itself.

The Manuals for the CBCL and TRF (Achenbach, 1991b, 1991c) provide evidence of construct validity for the CBCL and TRF syndromes in terms of significant correlations with syndrome scales derived from other instruments. However, the lack of instruments resembling the SCICA currently limits the possibilities for testing construct validity in this way. Testing the construct validity of the SCICA is therefore a task for future research. In the meantime, Chapter 8 presents correlations between comparable scales of the SCICA, CBCL, TRF, and DOF. The present chapter reports findings on the content validity of the SCICA items and criterion-related validity of the SCICA scale scores.

CONTENT VALIDITY OF SCICA ITEMS

Content validity refers to whether an instrument's content includes what it is intended to measure. As explained in Chapter 4, the SCICA items were based on CBCL and TRF items that were appropriate for the interview situation. The CBCL items were originally developed to describe problems that are of concern to parents and mental health workers. The CBCL items were derived from earlier research on child/adolescent psychiatric case histories (Achenbach, 1966), the clinical and research literature, and consultation with clinical and developmental psychologists, psychiatrists, and social workers. Pilot editions of the CBCL were tested at multiple sites and were revised on the basis of feedback from parents, paraprofessionals, and clinicians. The TRF includes 93 items derived from the CBCL, plus additional items appropriate to school settings. Nearly all items included in the 1991 CBCL and TRF problem scales significantly discriminated between referred and nonreferred children (Achenbach, 1991b, 1991c).

SCICA Item Scores for Referred Versus Nonreferred Children

To assess the ability of SCICA items to discriminate between referred and nonreferred children, we computed multiple regressions of each item score on referral status (scored *0* for nonreferred, *1* for referred), sex, age, and SES (scored on Hollingshead's, 1975, 9-step scale for parental occupation). Multiple regressions were performed using a forward entry procedure for predictors (SAS Institute, 1990), in the following order: referral status, sex, age, and SES.

The sample for the multiple regressions included 53 subjects aged 6-12 who were referred for mental health or special education services and 53 demographically similar nonreferred subjects who were recruited from local schools. The nonreferred subjects had not been referred for any mental health or special education services within the past year. The 106 subjects included 36 boys (68%) and 17 (32%) girls in each sample. The referred and nonreferred subjects were matched as closely as possible for age and SES. Of the 53 pairs, matching for age produced 24 pairs (45%) matched on exact year of age, 22 pairs (42%) within one year of age, and 7 pairs (13%) within two years of age.

The mean age was 8.6 (*s.d.* = 1.8) for the referred sample and 8.9 (*s.d.* = 1.5) for the nonreferred sample. Matching for SES produced 42 pairs (79%) matched exactly on Hollingshead's scale and 11 pairs (21%) matched within a 3-point difference in SES. The mean SES was 6.4 (*s.d.* = 1.8) for the referred sample and 6.8 (*s.d.* = 1.9) for the nonreferred sample.

Three observation items (118-120) and seven self-report items (220-226) were excluded from the multiple regression analyses because they were recent additions that had not been scored for all subjects. Fifteen observation items and 26 self-report items were also excluded because they were scored *0* for >103 (97%) of the 106 subjects.

Table 6-1 lists the 79 SCICA items that significantly (*p* <.05) discriminated between referred and nonreferred subjects. The table shows the effect sizes for referral status and the three demographic variables in terms of the semipartial r^2 obtained after partialling out prior independent variables in the forward entry procedure. According to Cohen's (1988) criteria, effects accounting for 2 to 13% of variance are considered small; effects accounting for 13 to 26% of variance are medium; and effects accounting for $\geq$26% of variance are large. To indicate possible chance effects, we have marked (superscript *e*) the number of nominally significant effects that could have arisen by chance in the analyses of each independent variable, based on a .05 *alpha* level and a .05 protection level for determining the number of chance findings. The effects marked as possibly due to chance were the smallest nominally significant effects for each variable (Sakoda et al., 1954).

The multiple regressions showed that referred subjects scored higher than nonreferred subjects on all 51 observation items and 25 of the 28 self-report items that showed significant (*p* <.05) effects of referral status. One item (*38. Fidgets*) showed a large effect of referral status, while 6 items showed medium effects, and 72 items showed small effects. Out of 185 tests of referral status, 14 nominally

Table 6-1
Percent of Variance Accounted for by Significant ($p<.05$) Effects of Referral Status, Sex, Age, and SES in SCICA Items

Item	Ref Stat[a]	Sex[b]	Age[c]	SES[d]
Observation Items				
3. Giggles	9	--	--	--
4. Acts too young	12	--	--	--
5. Apathetic	10	--	--	--
6. Argues	9	--	6^{Y}	--
7. Asks for feedback	10	--	--	6^{Le}
10. Irresponsible behavior	11	--	--	--
12. Bites fingernails	5	--	--	--
19. Complains of being bored	6	--	--	--
20. Complains of dizziness	12	--	--	4^{Ue}
21. Complains tasks too hard	9	--	--	--
23. Confused	5	--	--	--
26. Day-dreams	5	--	--	--
28. Demands met immediately	8	--	5^{Ye}	--
29. Difficulty with directions	5^{e}	--	--	--
32. Doesn't sit still	13	--	--	--
33. Easily distracted	12	--	--	--
35. Exaggerates	7	--	--	--
36. Explosive	6	--	--	--
38. Fidgets	26	--	--	--
40. Off task	9	--	--	--
44. Difficulty expressing self	4	4^{Fe}	--	--
46. Problems remembering facts	6	--	--	--
48. Impatient	12	--	--	--
51. Jokes too much	5	--	--	--
53. Lapses in attention	5	--	--	--
54. Laughs inappropriately	5	--	--	--
55. Leaves to go to toilet	7	--	--	--
61. Misbehaves, test limits	15	--	5^{Ye}	--
63. Needs coaxing	10	--	--	--
67. Out of seat	9	--	--	--
69. Perseverates	6	--	--	--

Table 6-1 (Continued)

Item	Ref Stat[a]	Sex[b]	Age[c]	SES[d]
70. Picks nose, skin	12	--	--	--
72. Refuses to talk	6	--	4^{Ye}	--
73. Reluctant to discuss feelings	16	--	--	--
76. Resistant	13	--	--	--
77. Says "don't know" a lot	8	--	--	--
79. Secretive	10	--	--	--
84. Shows off, silly	10	--	--	--
95. Mood changes	11	--	6^{Y}	--
97. Suspicious	5^{e}	--	--	--
98. Swears	4^{e}	--	--	--
99. Talks to self	4^{e}	--	--	--
104. Tremors	5	--	--	--
105. Manipulates	11	--	--	5^{Le}
107. Unhappy, sad, depressed	6	--	--	--
112. Wants to quit	10	--	--	--
114. Withdrawn	8	4^{Fe}	--	--
115. Careless	8	--	--	5^{Le}
116. Worries	4	--	--	--
117. Yawns	6	--	--	--
121. Other observed problems	4^{e}	--	--	--

Self-Report Items

Item	Ref Stat[a]	Sex[b]	Age[c]	SES[d]
130. Rpts disobedience at home	6	--	--	--
131. Rpts disobedience at school	7	5^{Me}	--	--
134. Rpts being lonely	5^{Ne}	--	--	--
135. Rpts harmed by parent	6	--	--	--
136. Rpts being punished	15	--	--	--
139. Rpts being shy	6^{Ne}	--	--	--
142. Rpts being treated unfairly at home	5^{e}	--	--	--
147. Rpts being unhappy, sad, depressed	8	--	--	--
152. Rpts crying a lot	6	7^{Fe}	--	--
158. Rpts difficulty learning	4^{e}	--	--	--

Table 6-1 (Continued)

Item	Ref Stat[a]	Sex[b]	Age[c]	SES[d]
159. Rpts disliking school/work	16	--	--	--
171. Rpts feeling worthless	6	--	4^{Oe}	--
172. Rpts getting hurt a lot	8	--	--	--
173. Rpts fighting	10	4^{Me}	--	--
175. Rpts hanging around others who get in trouble	6	--	4^{Oe}	--
177. Rpts hating parent	4	--	3^{Oe}	--
186. Rpts not getting along with parents	6	--	--	--
187. Rpts obsessive thoughts	3^e	--	--	--
188. Rpts attacking people	6	--	6^{Oe}	--
191. Rpts preferring younger kids	8	3^{Fe}	--	--
193. Rpts problems making friends	6	--	--	--
194. Rpts problems with school work	11	--	--	--
201. Rpts stealing outside home	4^e	--	--	--
205. Rpts temper tantrums	5	--	--	--
207. Rpts threatening people	4^e	--	--	--
208. Rpts trouble sleeping	4^e	6^{Fe}	--	4^{Ue}
214. Rpts worries	5^{Ne}	--	--	--
247. Other self-reported problems	9	--	--	--

Note. Analyses were multiple regressions of item scores on referral status, sex, age, and SES. The percent of variance accounted for by each independent variable is represented by the semipartial r^2 for that variable after partialling out any prior independent variables.
[a]Referred subjects scored higher, except items marked N.
[b]M = males scored higher; F = females scored higher.
[c]O = older subjects scored higher; Y = younger scored higher.
[d]U = upper SES scored higher; L = lower SES scored higher.
[e]Not significant when corrected for number of analyses.

significant effects may have been due to chance. These included 11 items on which referred subjects scored higher and the only 3 items on which nonreferred subjects scored higher.

Among the 79 items that showed significant effects of referral status, there were fewer effects of sex and SES than expected by chance. There were two more significant age effects than expected by chance, both reflecting higher scores for younger than older subjects.

CRITERION-RELATED VALIDITY OF SCICA SCALES

One of the main reasons for empirically deriving syndromes was the lack of a satisfactory taxonomy of child psychopathology. Although recent editions of the DSM have become more differentiated with respect to childhood disorders (American Psychiatric Association, 1980, 1987, 1994), the DSM's diagnostic categories have not been derived directly from data on children. There are similarities and statistical associations between several DSM categories and the syndromes derived from the CBCL, TRF, and YSR (Biederman et al., 1993; Edelbrock & Costello, 1988; Gould, Bird, & Jaramillo, 1993; Weinstein, Noam, Grimes, Stone, & Schwab-Stone, 1990). Nevertheless, the DSM categories are not operationally defined according to any particular assessment procedures.

In lieu of better validated diagnostic criteria, we have used actual referral for mental health services to test the criterion-related validity of our empirically derived scales. We recognize that referral for mental health services is not an infallible criterion of need for help. Some youths in our referred sample may not have needed professional help, whereas some in our nonreferred sample may have needed help. Yet, as detailed elsewhere (Achenbach & Edelbrock, 1981), actual referral seemed as ecologically valid as any other practical alternative for testing criterion-related validity.

Scale Scores of Referred Versus Nonreferred Children

To test the differences between scale scores obtained by our matched samples of referred versus nonreferred subjects ($N = 106$), we performed 2 x 2 ANCOVAs treating referral status and sex as independent variables and SES (scored on Hollingshead's 9-point scale) as the covariate. Using GLM procedures (SAS Institute, 1990), separate ANCOVAs were performed on each of the eight SCICA syndromes, Internalizing, Externalizing, total Observation score, and total Self-Report score. The ANCOVAs were performed on raw scores to avoid the truncation of low scores that occurs with T scores (see Chapter 4).

Referred subjects scored significantly higher ($p < .05$) than nonreferred subjects on all SCICA scales, except the Anxious scale ($p = .09$). Of the 12 tests of referral status, two significant effects showing the smallest F values could be due to chance (Strange and Internalizing). Effects of SES, sex, and interactions between sex and referral status did not exceed chance expectations. To provide a common metric for displaying scores for the matched referred and nonreferred samples, Figure 6-1 shows their mean T scores for the eight SCICA syndromes, while Figure 6-2 shows their mean T scores for Internalizing, Externalizing, total Observation score, and total Self-Report score. Appendix C lists the means and standard deviations of raw scores and T scores on all SCICA scales for the same samples.

Multiple Regressions of Scale Scores

To further assess the effects of referral status and the demographic variables on SCICA scale scores, we computed multiple regressions of each scale score on referral status, sex, age, and SES, entered in this order. Table 6-2 shows the effect size for each variable in terms of the semipartial r^2 obtained after partialling out any prior independent variables in the forward entry procedure. The two nominally

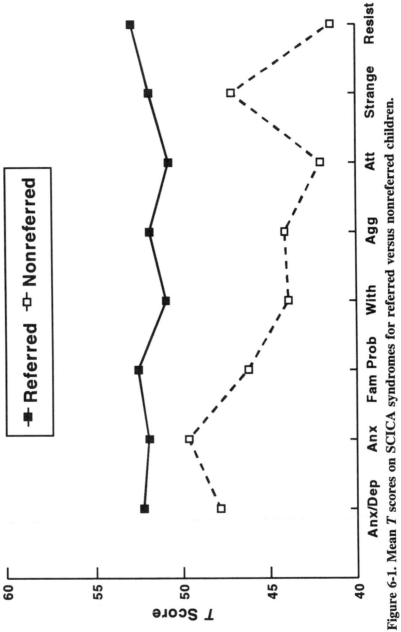

Figure 6-1. Mean *T* scores on SCICA syndromes for referred versus nonreferred children.

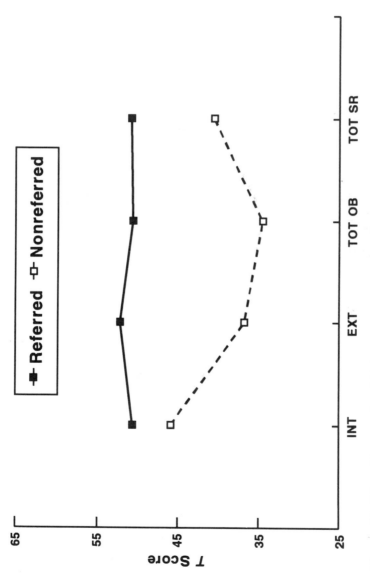

Figure 6-2. Mean *T* scores for SCICA Internalizing, Externalizing, and total scores for referred versus nonreferred children.

VALIDITY

Table 6-2
Percent of Variance Accounted for by Significant (p <.05) Effects of Referral Status, Sex, Age, and SES in SCICA Scale Scores for Matched Referred and Nonreferred Samples

Scale	Ref. Stat.[a]	Sex[b]	Age[c]	SES[d]
Anxious/Depressed[SR]	8	--	5[O]	--
Anxious[OB]	--[e]	--	5[Of]	--
Family Problems[SR]	11	--	--	--
Withdrawn[OB]	11	--	4[Yf]	--
Aggressive Behavior[SR]	14	5[Mf]	5[O]	--
Attention Problems[OB]	23	--	--	--
Strange[OB]	5[f]	--	--	--
Resistant[OB]	28	--	4[Y]	--
Internalizing	7[f]	--	7[O]	3[Lf]
Externalizing	31	--	--	--
Total Observations	42	--	--	--
Total Self-Reports	22	--	7[O]	--

Note. Analyses were multiple regressions of raw scale scores on referral status, sex, age, and SES. The percent of variance accounted for by each independent variable is represented by the semipartial r^2 for that variable after partialling out any prior independent variables.
[a]All scores were higher for referred than nonreferred subjects.
[b]M = males scored higher.
[c]O = older subjects scored higher; Y = younger scored higher.
[d]L = lower SES subjects scored higher.
[e]For Anxious, referred scored higher than nonreferred at p = .07, accounting for 2% of variance.
[f]Not significant when corrected for number of analyses.

significant findings likely to occur by chance are marked by superscript *f*.

Referred subjects obtained significantly (p <.05) higher scores on all SCICA scales, except Anxious (p = .07). The effects of referral status were large for Resistant (28% of variance), Externalizing (31%), total Observation score (42%), and total Self-Report score (22%). Effects were medium for Attention Problems (23%) and Aggressive Behavior (14%), and small for the remaining four scales (5 to 11%). The nine significant ($p < .05$) effects of the three demographic variables were small (3 to 7% of variance). Four of these were likely due to chance. A significant sex effect was found only for Aggressive Behavior, with boys scoring higher than girls, but this was likely to be a chance finding. Five significant nonchance age effects showed that older subjects scored higher on Anxious/Depressed, Aggressive Behavior, Internalizing, and total Self-Report, whereas younger subjects scored higher on Resistant. There were no significant nonchance effects of SES.

Discriminant Analyses

We performed discriminant analyses to determine which weighted combinations of SCICA scale scores best differentiated referred from nonreferred subjects. Three sets of discriminant analyses were performed for the matched referred and nonreferred samples ($N = 106$), using the following candidate predictors: *(1)* the eight SCICA syndromes; *(2)* Internalizing and Externalizing; and *(3)* the total Observation and total Self-Report scores.

Discriminant analyses selectively weight predictors to maximize their collective associations with the criterion groups being analyzed. The weighting process makes use of characteristics of the sample that may differ from other samples. To avoid overestimating the accuracy of the classification obtained by the discriminant analyses, it is therefore necessary to correct for "shrinkage" in the classification accuracy that would occur when discriminant weights derived in one sample are applied to a new sample. To correct for shrinkage, we employed a "jackknife" procedure whereby separate discriminant functions were computed with a different subject held out of the sample each time (SAS Institute, 1990). These discriminant functions were cross-validated by testing the accuracy of their predictions for each of the "hold-out" subjects. The percentage of correct predictions was then averaged across all the hold-out subjects. The resulting cross-validated predictions are presented below.

The weighted combination of the eight SCICA syndromes correctly classified 77.4% of cases as referred (sensitivity) and 86.8% as nonreferred (specificity). The overall misclassification rate was 17.9%, with 13.2% of nonreferred cases incorrectly classified as "referred" (false positives), and 22.6% of referred cases incorrectly classified as "nonreferred" (false negatives). The overall misclassification rate of 17.9% for the SCICA syndromes was comparable to the 17.7% misclassification rate obtained using the borderline clinical cutpoints for the CBCL competence and syndrome scales (Achenbach, 1991b).

The weighted combination of the SCICA Internalizing and Externalizing scores correctly classified 66% of cases as referred and 83% as nonreferred, with an overall misclassification rate of 25.5%, which was higher than the misclassification rate for the eight syndromes. The weighted combination of the total Observation and Self-Report scores produced classification rates comparable to those for the eight syndromes, with 79.3% correctly classified as referred, 86.8% correctly classified as nonreferred, and an overall misclassification rate of 17.0%.

SUMMARY

This chapter presented several kinds of evidence for the validity of the SCICA scores. *Content validity* was tested for 185 SCICA items scored as present for at least 3% of 106 demographically matched referred and nonreferred subjects. Of these, 76 items were scored significantly higher for referred than nonreferred subjects. Item *38. Fidgets* showed a large effect of referral status, 6 items showed medium effects, and the remaining items showed small effects.

Criterion-related validity was supported by the ability of the SCICA scale scores to discriminate between referred and nonreferred subjects. Referred subjects scored significantly higher than nonreferred subjects on all but one (Anxious) of the eight syndromes, as well as Internalizing, Externalizing, total Observation score, and total Self-Report score. Large effects of referral status were found for the Resistant syndrome, Externalizing, and total Observation score, accounting for 28 to 42% of variance. After adjusting for the number of chance findings, there were no significant effects of sex or SES, and only five small effects of age. A weighted combination of the eight SCICA syndromes yielded 77.4% sensitivity and 86.8% specificity, for an overall misclassification rate of 17.9%. A weighted combination of the total Observation and total Self-Report scores yielded 79.3% sensitivity and 86.8% specificity, for an overall misclassification rate of 17.0%.

Chapter 7
Relations Between Pre-1994 and 1994 Scales

This chapter highlights similarities and differences between the pre-1994 SCIC and the 1994 SCICA scales, plus the correlations between the counterpart scales.

The construction of the 1994 scales was described in Chapter 4. Like the pre-1994 syndrome scales, the 1994 syndrome scales were derived from separate principal components/varimax analyses of Observation and Self-Report item scores averaged from ratings by interviewers and videotape observers. The 1994 sample included the pre-1994 sample of 108 clinically referred children, plus an additional 60 referred children, for a total N of 168.

The overall strategy of scale construction was similar, but the larger 1994 sample yielded syndromes that differed somewhat from the pre-1994 syndromes. Because of the larger derivation sample, the 1994 syndromes are likely to be more accurate representations of the relations among items.

The T scores for the 1994 scales were based on ratings of 237 referred children, compared to 108 for the pre-1994 scales. In assigning the 1994 T scores, we gave equal weight to the distributions of raw scores obtained from girls and boys, as described in Chapter 4. The larger sample and equal weighting of scores provide a firmer basis for judging how individual boys' and girls' scores on each scale compare with those of referred children who have been interviewed with the SCICA.

Additional innovations include the following:

1. Normalized T scores were based on the midpoints between percentiles of the raw score distributions.

2. Syndrome scales were truncated at $T = 38$, rather than $T = 40$ as on the pre-1994 scales.

3. No items are included in more than one syndrome scale, nor in both the Internalizing and Externalizing groupings.

4. On the hand-scored profile, Internalizing and Externalizing scores can be calculated by summing syndrome scale scores without having to sum individual items from the Observation and Self-Report Forms.

STATISTICAL RELATIONS BETWEEN PRE-1994 AND 1994 SCALES

Six of the 1994 syndromes have titles that are similar to those of pre-1994 syndromes. Of the remaining two 1994 syndromes, the 21-item Anxious/Depressed syndrome includes 13 items from the pre-1994 Inept syndrome, but also other items indicative of anxiety and depression, such as *141. Reports being too fearful or anxious; 147. Reports being unhappy, sad, or depressed; 160. Reports fear of making mistakes; 164. Reports feeling guilty;* and *214. Reports worrying.* As shown in Table 7-1, the correlation of .90 between the 1994 Anxious/Depressed syndrome and the pre-1994 Inept syndrome indicates that they both tap a similar construct. The label Anxious/Depressed was chosen for the 1994 version in view of the addition of several items indicative of affective problems, plus the fact that 9 of the 21 items have counterparts on the CBCL Anxious/Depressed syndrome.

The only 1994 syndrome that lacks a clear pre-1994 counterpart is the one designated as Strange. The highest

Table 7-1
Pearson Correlations Between Raw Scores
for Pre-1994 and 1994 Scales

1994 Scale	Correlation
Anxious/Depressed[a]	.90
Anxious	.95
Family Problems	.79
Withdrawn[b]	.99
Aggressive Behavior	.96
Attention Problems[c]	.86
Strange[d]	.55
Resistant	.95
Internalizing	.96
Externalizing	.49

Note. Correlations were computed in a sample consisting of 237 referred and 53 nonreferred children. All *r*s were significant at *p* <.001. Total Observation and Self-Report scales are omitted, because the 1994 and pre-1994 versions were identical for this sample. [a]The closest pre-1994 counterpart was titled Inept. [b]Pre-1994 version was titled Withdrawn-Depressed. [c]Pre-1994 version was titled Inattentive-Hyperactive. [d]The 1994 Strange scale had no clear pre-1994 counterpart; its highest correlation was with the pre-1994 Inattentive-Hyperactive scale.

loading items on this syndrome were *92. Strange ideas* (loading = .59) and *30. Disjointed or tangential conversation* (loading = .53). Other items included *17. Can't get mind off certain thoughts; obsessions* (loading = .49) and *91. Strange behavior* (loading = .36). This syndrome reflects a pattern of relatively rare and bizarre problems that may not have been detected previously because of the smaller size of the derivation sample. As shown in Table 7-1, the Strange syndrome's highest correlation (.55) was with the pre-1994 Inattentive-Hyperactive syndrome. This reflects the fact that children who score high on the Strange syndrome also tend to have problems with attention and hyperactivity. In fact, as shown in Appendix D, the 1994 Strange syndrome correlated higher with the 1994 Attention Problems syndrome than with any other 1994 syndrome ($r = .44$ in the referred sample; $r = .57$ in the nonreferred sample). Nevertheless, many children may score high on the Attention Problems syndrome without necessarily scoring high on the Strange syndrome, and vice versa.

As Table 7-1 shows, the six syndromes that were given similar labels in the pre-1994 and 1994 analyses yielded correlations ranging from .79 for Family Problems to .99 for Withdrawn (whose pre-1994 version was designated as Withdrawn-Depressed).

The correlation of .96 between the pre-1994 and 1994 Internalizing scales indicates that they reflect similar characteristics. The considerably lower correlation of .49 between the pre-1994 and 1994 Externalizing scales reflects the fact that only the Aggressive and Family Problems syndromes loaded on the pre-1994 Externalizing factor. By contrast, the Aggressive, Attention Problems, Strange, and Resistant syndromes all loaded on the 1994 Externalizing factor, whereas the Family Problems syndrome did not. The 1994 Externalizing grouping thus encompasses a much broader range of phenomena than its pre-1994 counterpart.

The scores obtained on the pre-1994 syndromes, Internalizing, and Externalizing are not directly comparable with those on the 1994 versions, because of changes in the items that comprise each scale. A particular score on a pre-1994 scale is thus unlikely to have the same meaning as that score on the 1994 counterpart scale.

Correlations between pre-1994 and 1994 total Observation and Self-Report scores were 1.00, because they comprised the same items. The few new items added to the

1994 Observation and Self-Report Forms had not been scored for enough subjects to warrant including them in the computation of correlations.

SUMMARY

This chapter highlighted similarities and differences between the pre-1994 SCIC and the 1994 SCICA scales, plus the correlations between the counterpart scales.

The overall strategy of scale construction was similar, but the 1994 analyses and assignment of T scores were based on considerably larger samples. Scores from boys and girls were equally weighted in assigning T scores.

Innovations in the 1994 scales include: normalized T scores based on midpoint percentiles; syndrome scales truncated at $T = 38$; no items included on more than one scale; and easier hand-scoring of Internalizing and Externalizing.

Among the six syndromes having similar titles, the pre-1994 versions correlated .79 to .99 with the 1994 versions. In addition, the 1994 Anxious/Depressed syndrome correlated .90 with the pre-1994 syndrome designated as Inept, indicating that they both tap a similar construct. The 1994 Internalizing scale correlated .96 with its pre-1994 counterpart. However, the two versions of the Externalizing scales correlated only .49, reflecting the major changes in the composition of this grouping.

Because of the changes in syndrome scales, Internalizing, and Externalizing, a particular score on the pre-1994 version of a syndrome is not directly comparable to any particular score on the 1994 version. Nevertheless, the high correlations between most pre-1994 scales and their 1994 counterparts indicate that correlational and other analyses involving the relative magnitude of scores within particular distributions would produce similar results on most of the corresponding pre-1994 and 1994 scales.

Chapter 8
Relations to Other
Assessment Procedures

The SCICA is designed to function as one component of a multiaxial empirically based approach to assessment, as outlined in Chapter 1. Other components that most directly parallel the SCICA include the CBCL, TRF, YSR, and DOF. Fifty items of the SCICA Observation Form and 81 items of the Self-Report Form are based on CBCL items. In addition to the CBCL-based items that have counterparts on the TRF, an additional 12 Observation items and 6 Self-Report items are based on TRF items. Ninety-four SCICA items drawn from the CBCL or TRF also have counterparts on the YSR, while 84 have counterparts on the DOF.

Although 149 SCICA items have counterparts on one or more of the other instruments, the precise wording of items, the target assessment period, the informants, and the assessment conditions all vary among the instruments. As a consequence, the assessment of a particular problem by one procedure cannot substitute for assessment by the other procedures. Instead, multiple procedures are needed to detect similarities and differences between problems reported for the same individual by different informants. Although not all sources of data are relevant or feasible in all cases, the use of more than one source is usually necessary for comprehensive clinical assessment of children and adolescents.

Chapter 10 illustrates some ways in which multiple sources are used in particular cases. To provide an overview of the levels of agreement found between scale scores obtained from different informants, this chapter presents correlations between the SCICA scales and CBCL, TRF, and

DOF scales. Because the YSR is designed for ages 11-18, it is less relevant to the SCICA scales for ages 6-12 than are the CBCL, TRF, and DOF.

RELATIONS BETWEEN
THE SCICA AND CBCL

We computed Pearson correlations between SCICA raw scale scores and raw scale scores from CBCLs that were completed by parents within 2 months of the SCICA. The subjects were 158 clinically referred children, plus 34 nonreferred children who were drawn from the sample described in Chapter 6, for a total $N = 192$. There were 132 boys and 60 girls, with Ns ranging from 13 to 43 subjects at each age from 6 to 12.

Although there were many significant correlations between SCICA and CBCL scales, we will focus primarily on the highest correlation that each SCICA scale had with a CBCL syndrome scale. Table 8-1 displays these correlations, plus the highest correlation that each SCICA scale had with the CBCL Internalizing, Externalizing, or total problem score. Except as noted, the correlations in Table 8-1 were significant at $p \leq .01$. Superscript b indicates those that were most likely to have reached $p \leq .01$ by chance among the 132 correlations that were computed (12 SCICA scales x 11 CBCL scales). Ranging from .19 to .48, the correlations in Table 8-1 are commensurate with those found in meta-analyses of correlations between ratings by different types of informants seeing children under different conditions in many studies (Achenbach et al., 1987).

The four SCICA syndromes that bear names corresponding to CBCL syndromes all correlated higher with the corresponding CBCL syndrome than with any other CBCL syndrome, as follows: Anxious/Depressed, $r = .23$; Withdrawn, $r = .35$; Aggressive Behavior, $r = .43$; and Attention Problems, $r = .37$. Of the other four SCICA syndromes, the highest correlation for Family Problems was with the CBCL

Table 8-1

Pearson Correlations Between SCICA and CBCL[a] Problem Scales

SCICA Scales	CBCL Scales								
	With-drawn	Somatic Compl.	Anx/ Dep.	Social Probs.	Att. Probs.	Aggres-sive	Inter-nalizing	Exter-nalizing	Total Probs.
Anx/Dep.			.23				.24		
Anxious						(-.15)	.22	(-.15)	
Family Probs.		.24							
Withdrawn	.35								.19[b]
Aggressive						.43		.44	.33
Attention Probs.					.37				
Strange				.26					.21
Resistant				.41				.36	
Internalizing		.19[b]					.21		
Externalizing				.48				.45	.45
Total OB				.43					.41
Total SR			.29				.33		

Note. N = 192, including 158 clinically referred and 34 nonreferred children whose parents completed the CBCL within 2 months of the SCICA. Ages were 6-12; 132 were boys, 60 were girls. The rs are the highest that each SCICA scale had with a CBCL syndrome and with a CBCL Internalizing, Externalizing, or total problem scale. All rs in the table were p ≤.01, except those in parentheses, which were p <.05.
[a]The CBCL Thought Problems and Delinquent Behavior scales are omitted, because no SCICA scale had a higher r with either of them than with another CBCL syndrome.
[b]When corrected for the 132 rs computed between 12 SCICA scales and 11 CBCL scales, r = .19 was among the 5 p ≤.01 rs that could be attributed to chance.

Somatic Complaints syndrome ($r = .24$), while the highest correlations for both the Strange and Resistant syndromes were with the CBCL Social Problems syndrome ($r = .26$ and .41, respectively). The significant correlation between the SCICA Family Problems syndrome and the CBCL Somatic Complaints syndrome probably reflects the two somatic items (headaches and stomachaches) on the Family Problems syndrome. This correlation and the loading of the two somatic items on the syndrome characterized mainly by family problems suggest a pattern of associations between somatic complaints and the types of self-reported stress characterizing the other items of the Family Problems syndrome. The significant correlations of the CBCL Social Problems syndrome with both the Strange and Resistant syndromes suggest that the interpersonal difficulties reflected in parents' ratings of Social Problems tend to be manifested in the interview situation in terms of the Strange and Resistant syndromes.

The SCICA Anxious syndrome had no correlations that were significant at $p \leq .01$ with any CBCL scales. However, the Anxious syndrome correlated $-.15$ ($p < .05$) with both the CBCL Aggressive Behavior and Externalizing scales. These negative correlations indicate a small tendency for children who display externalizing behavior problems with their parents to show little anxiety during the interview. Moreover, the SCICA Aggressive Behavior syndrome's correlations with the CBCL Aggressive Behavior syndrome ($r = .43$) and with the CBCL Externalizing scale ($r = .44$) indicate moderate consistency between reports of aggressive behavior by parents and children's self-reports during the interview.

In addition to correlating with CBCL problem scales, most SCICA scales had significant (negative) correlations with CBCL competence scales. The SCICA Resistant, Externalizing, and total Observation scales had their largest correlations with the CBCL total competence scale ($rs = -.36, -.37,$ and $-.41$, respectively). The SCICA Withdrawn,

Aggressive Behavior, Attention Problems, and total Self-Report scales had their largest correlations with the CBCL School scale (r = -.31, -.29, -.34, and -.26, respectively). After excluding the number of correlations expected to be significant by chance, the remaining SCICA scales did not have any correlations with CBCL competence scales that were significant at $p \leq .01$.

RELATIONS BETWEEN THE SCICA AND TRF

Following our procedure for testing relations between SCICA and CBCL scales, we computed Pearson correlations between SCICA raw scale scores and raw scale scores from TRFs that were completed by teachers within 2 months of the SCICA. The subjects were 147 clinically referred children, plus 33 nonreferred children drawn from the same sample as the CBCLs, for a total $N = 180$. There were 126 boys and 54 girls, with Ns ranging from 9 to 38 at each age from 6 to 12.

As with the CBCL, we will focus primarily on the highest correlation that each SCICA scale had with a TRF syndrome. Table 8-2 displays these correlations, plus the highest correlation that each SCICA scale had with the TRF Internalizing, Externalizing, or total problem score.

The SCICA Withdrawn, Aggressive Behavior, and Attention Problems syndromes correlated higher with their namesake TRF syndromes than with any other TRF syndromes (rs = .19, .44, and .41, respectively). The SCICA Anxious/Depressed syndrome did not correlate significantly with the TRF Anxious/Depressed syndrome, but it correlated .22 with the TRF Withdrawn syndrome.

The SCICA Resistant syndrome correlated .52 with both the TRF Aggressive Behavior syndrome and Externalizing scale, while the SCICA Externalizing scale correlated .54 with both these TRF scales, plus the TRF total problem score. The SCICA Strange syndrome correlated .33 with the TRF Thought Problems syndrome, while the SCICA Family

Table 8-2
Pearson Correlations Between SCICA and TRF[a] Problem Scales

SCICA Scales	TRF Scales								
	With-drawn	Somatic Compl.	Thought Probs.	Att. Probs.	Delin-quent	Aggres-sive	Inter-nalizing	Exter-nalizing	Total Probs.
Anx/Dep.	.22								
Anxious					(-.17)			(-.15)	
Family Probs.		.20							
Withdrawn	.19[b]								
Aggressive						.44		.45	.41
Attention Probs.				.41					
Strange			.33						.23
Resistant						.52		.52	
Internalizing	.20								
Externalizing						.54		.54	.54
Total OB						.39			
Total SR	.26						.19[b]		.41

Note. $N = 180$, including 147 clinically referred and 33 nonreferred children whose teachers completed the TRF within 2 months of the SCICA. Ages were 6-12; 126 were boys, 54 were girls. The *r*s are the highest that each SCICA scale had with a TRF syndrome and with a TRF Internalizing, Externalizing, or total problem scale. All *r*s in the table were $p \leq .01$, except those in parentheses, which were $p < .05$.

[a]The TRF Anxious/Depressed and Social Problems scales are omitted, because no SCICA scale had a higher *r* with them than with another TRF syndrome.

[b]When corrected for the 132 *r*s computed between 12 SCICA scales and 11 TRF scales, $r = .19$ was among the 5 $p \leq .01$ *r*s that could be attributed to chance.

Problems syndrome correlated .20 with the TRF Somatic Complaints syndrome. This was similar to the correlation of .24 found between the SCICA Family Problems and CBCL Somatic Complaints syndromes. Also similar to the correlations found between the SCICA and CBCL, the SCICA Anxious syndrome correlated -.15 with the TRF Externalizing scale ($p < .05$). Although the negative correlations were small, both teacher and parent reports thus indicate that externalizing behavior outside the interview is associated with low levels of anxiety, as well as with high levels of externalizing behavior, in the interview.

The SCICA Aggressive Behavior, Attention Problems, Externalizing, and total Observation scores all correlated negatively ($p < .01$) with the TRF academic performance score, all four TRF adaptive items, and the total adaptive behavior score. The SCICA Resistant and total Self-Report scores also correlated negatively ($p < .01$) with 5 of these 6 TRF scores. The SCICA Externalizing score yielded the largest correlations, including -.50 with the TRF score for how appropriately the child behaves and -.43 for the TRF total adaptive score. The correlations of the SCICA Internalizing score and the other SCICA syndromes with the TRF adaptive scores did not reach $p \leq .01$. Teachers' reports of poor adaptive functioning were thus associated primarily with externalizing problems in the interview situation.

RELATIONS BETWEEN THE SCICA AND DOF

The DOF is designed to obtain samples of behavior observed in group settings such as classrooms. In using the DOF, an observer writes a narrative description of the target child's behavior and interactions with others over a 10-minute period. At the end of each minute, the observer scores the child as being on-task or not, yielding a score of 0 to 10 for on-task behavior over the 10-minute observation period. Based on the 10-minute narrative description of the child's behavior, the observer rates 96 problem items, using scores ranging from 0 to 3 that are defined like those on the SCICA. The observer's ratings are summed to yield scale scores for six empirically derived syndromes, Internalizing, Externalizing, and total problems. Multiple 10-minute samples are obtained and averaged to provide scores that are more representative than a single sample would be.

We computed Pearson correlations between SCICA and DOF scale scores obtained by 75 referred children, based on averaging three 10-minute observations of classroom behavior for each child. There were 48 boys and 27 girls, with Ns ranging from 9 to 17 at each age from 6 to 11.

Beside the five expected to reach $p \leq .01$ by chance among the 120 correlations (12 SCICA scales x 10 DOF scales), five others were significant at $p < .01$. All of these involved the DOF Aggressive and Externalizing scales, which correlated from .35 to .46 with the SCICA Attention Problems, Resistant, and Externalizing scales. (The SCICA and DOF Aggressive scales also correlated .33, $p = .004$, but this was one of the five significant correlations that was most likely to occur by chance.) There was thus moderate consistency between externalizing kinds of problems observed in the classroom and interview situations.

Separate analyses for each sex showed more significant SCICA x DOF correlations for girls than for boys or for both sexes combined, whereas the SCICA's correlations with the CBCL and TRF were generally similar for both sexes. Even though only 27 girls were scored on the DOF, nine correlations were significant at $p < .01$, beside the five that were most likely to be significant by chance. The correlations for girls ranged up to .61 between the DOF Aggressive scale and the SCICA Attention Problems scale. In addition, there were large negative correlations between the DOF Aggressive scale and the SCICA Anxious/Depressed, Internalizing, and total Self-Report scores (rs = -.60, -.53, and -.62, respectively). Although replication in larger samples is needed, it thus appears that behavior observed in classrooms is related to problems observed and reported in interviews more strongly for girls than boys.

SUMMARY

Correlations of SCICA scales with CBCL and TRF scales were commensurate with those found in other studies of associations between different sources of data concerning children's problems. The SCICA syndromes that bear the same names as CBCL and TRF syndromes had their highest correlations with all four of their CBCL namesakes and three of their four TRF namesakes. Externalizing scales tended to yield the highest correlations between the SCICA and the CBCL, TRF, and DOF. CBCL competence scores and TRF adaptive and academic performance scores had significant negative correlations with several SCICA scales, especially externalizing scales. Although the CBCL and TRF yielded generally similar findings for both sexes, significant correlations between the DOF and SCICA were more numerous for girls than for boys.

Chapter 9
Applications of the SCICA

The SCICA is designed for use in clinical assessment, research, and training. By providing a standardized interview that can be used for different purposes in diverse settings, we hope to advance the integration of clinical practice, research, and training with one another. Such integration can bring research into closer contact with the needs of clinical practice and can help practice and training benefit more directly from the fruits of research. In this chapter, we outline some of the ways in which the SCICA can be used.

APPLICATIONS TO CLINICAL ASSESSMENT

The SCICA is intended to contribute to clinical assessment by providing greater standardization of interview procedures and more explicit, reliable, and differentiated assessment data for each child. Neither an interview nor any other procedure can provide all the data needed for comprehensive clinical evaluations of children. Instead, the value of interviews depends on their ability to contribute data that are not more easily obtainable in other ways, to assess children's views of their own functioning, and to facilitate a therapeutic alliance in preparation for possible treatment. Interviews can also sample behavior and emotional responses relevant to the choice of therapy. We view the SCICA as one form of direct assessment that may also include other assessment procedures, such as observations in natural settings and tests of personality and self-concept. The direct assessment of the child, in turn, constitutes one of five sources of data that may be relevant to the clinical assessment of most children. Other sources include parents, teachers, cognitive tests, and physical assessment, as discussed in Chapter 1.

Mental Health Contexts

Because the SCICA is designed to blend comfortably with prevailing clinical practice, it can serve as the initial assessment interview for outpatient and inpatient mental health services. To keep the interviewer's judgments from being unduly influenced by data from other sources, it is desirable for the interviewer to be blind with respect to the referral complaints and other background information about the child. If feasible, the six CBCL or TRF problem items that the interviewer is to inquire about should be entered on the SCICA Protocol by an assistant prior to administering the SCICA. If this is not feasible, the clinician should arrange the assessment procedures in a sequence suitable for the situation.

Beside providing the basis for scoring the Self-Report and Observation items, the SCICA enables the child to become acquainted with the clinician and the clinician to judge the child's potential suitability for different treatment modalities. The item scores, scale scores on the SCICA Profile, and the profile pattern can be compared with data from other sources, such as the CBCL and TRF, to identify similarities and differences between the problems reported by different informants. Together with the developmental history, family background data, and test findings, these can be used to decide whether intervention is warranted and, if so, what sort of intervention. Following either an intervention or a period without an intervention, the SCICA, CBCL, and/or TRF can be readministered to evaluate change from the initial assessment. Figure 9-1 outlines a sequence of this sort.

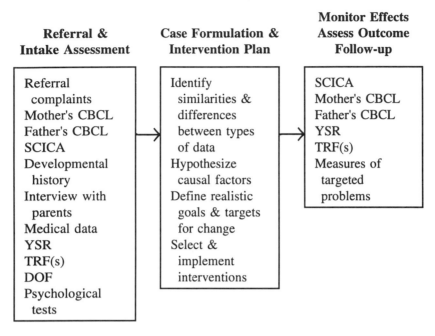

Fig. 9-1. Schematic sequence for assessment of children referred for mental health services.

School Contexts

The SCICA can be used with other assessment procedures for comprehensive special education evaluations mandated by the Individuals with Disabilities Education Act (IDEA; Public Law 101-476, 1990). It is especially helpful for determining whether a child qualifies for special education services under the IDEA category of Serious Emotional Disturbance (SED), which is defined as follows:

> (i) The term means a condition exhibiting one or more of the following characteristics over a long period of time and to a marked degree, which adversely affects educational performance:
>
> A. An inability to learn which cannot be explained by intellectual, sensory, or other health factors;

B. An inability to build or maintain satisfactory interpersonal relationships with peers and teachers;

C. Inappropriate types of behavior or feelings under normal circumstances;

D. A general pervasive mood of unhappiness or depression; or

E. A tendency to develop physical symptoms or fears associated with personal or school problems;

(ii) The term includes children who are schizophrenic. The term does not include children who are socially maladjusted unless it is determined that they have a serious emotional disturbance.

States vary in their interpretations of the IDEA definition of SED. Some states include externalizing behavior disorders in their criteria for SED, while other states exclude such behavior disorders. However, research shows that externalizing and internalizing problems often co-occur in referred and nonreferred children (McConaughy & Skiba, 1993). For children exhibiting either internalizing or externalizing problems, the SCICA can be useful for direct assessment of the pattern and severity of problems for comparison with parent and teacher reports.

Table 9-1 outlines relations between the IDEA criteria for SED and the empirically based syndromes of the SCICA, CBCL, TRF, YSR, and DOF. The table lists the syndromes of each instrument next to the SED characteristics that they most clearly represent. The table also shows how scores and scales of the various instruments can provide evidence of the three qualifying conditions of a *long period of time, marked degree,* and *adversely affects educational performance.* Similar applications of our empirically based measures to SED criteria have been described elsewhere (McConaughy, 1993a, 1993b; McConaughy, Mattison, & Peterson, 1994; McConaughy & Ritter, in press).

Table 9-1

Relations between IDEA Criteria for SED and Empirically Based Syndromes

IDEA Criteria for SED[a]	SCICA	CBCL, TRF, & YSR	DOF
Inability to learn	Attention Problems	Attention Problems	Withdrawn-Inattentive
Inability to build or maintain relationships	Withdrawn	Social Problems Withdrawn	--
Inappropriate types of behavior or feelings	Aggressive Behavior Resistant Strange	Aggressive Behavior Thought Problems	Nervous-Obsessive Attention-Demanding Aggress., Hyper.
General unhappiness	Anxious/Depressed	Anxious/Depressed	Depressed
Tendency to develop physical symptoms or fears	Anxious Anxious/Depressed	Anxious/Depressed Somatic Complaints	--
Long period of time	Follow-up evaluations	Follow-up evaluations	Follow-up eval.
Marked degree	High scores for total Observations, total Self-Reports, Internaliz., Externaliz., or syndromes	High scores for total probs., Internaliz., Externaliz., or syndromes	High scores for total prob., Internaliz., Externaliz., or syndromes
Adversely affects educational performance	Low SCICA achievement test scores	Low scores for CBCL School, TRF Academic Performance, and/or TRF Adaptive Funct.	Low on-task score

[a]Individuals with Disabilities Education Act criteria for Serious Emotional Disturbance.

If referred pupils show deviance on scales of several instruments relevant to the SED criteria, these results can be added to other evidence gathered by a Basic Staffing Team (BST) to justify eligibility for special education services. Unlike the CBCL, TRF, YSR, and DOF, the SCICA does not have clinical cutpoints. However, high scores on the SCICA scales indicate deviance in comparison to the mean scores for referred and nonreferred children listed in Appendix C. For evaluations of SED in 6-12-year olds, the SCICA may be more appropriate than projective tests or self-administered personality tests which usually require more advanced cognitive development and language skills. Chapter 10 presents two case illustrations in which data from the SCICA, CBCL, TRF, and YSR were used to determine whether children met IDEA criteria for SED.

Forensic Contexts

Interviews with children are often required in court-related evaluations. Examples include evaluation for custody and placement decisions and evaluations following stressful experiences such as abuse or family disruption. As in mental health and school contexts, interviews for forensic purposes should be used in conjunction with other assessment procedures. The standardized SCICA Protocol, scoring forms, and SCICA Profile may be especially useful for presentation in court, if confidentiality is properly protected. The SCICA provides an explicit structure that is understandable by court personnel and that parallels the CBCL, TRF, and YSR with which the SCICA is typically used. Findings from the SCICA can be more systematically compared with reports from parents or parent surrogates, such as foster parents, and with reports by teachers, than can findings from traditional interviews. Comparisons might indicate, for example, that a report by a particular informant disagrees with data from all the other sources. Such a finding would argue for especially close scrutiny of that informant's knowledge, judgment, or candor regarding the child.

Reassessments are sometimes needed to evaluate possible changes in a child's functioning, such as after a trial placement with a parent or in a foster home. When the SCICA is repeated for each successive evaluation, the SCICA Profiles can be compared across the evaluations to identify changes in specific items, scale scores, profile patterns, and total problem scores. If CBCLs, TRFs, YSRs, and/or DOFs are obtained for each evaluation, they can likewise be compared to identify changes as seen by different informants. As with initial evaluations, such comparisons make it possible to explicitly document differences between assessments and between sources.

APPLICATIONS TO RESEARCH

The SCICA can be used for many of the same research purposes as our other empirically based assessment instruments, as outlined in the Manuals for the CBCL, TRF, and YSR. However, because it requires a skilled interviewer and 60 to 90 minutes with the subject in a private interview, large scale applications may not be as feasible as with the CBCL, TRF, and YSR. Nevertheless, the SCICA can be used in large scale studies when intensive face-to-face assessments are needed for either entire samples or subsamples. In many smaller studies, the 60- to 90-minute administration time should be quite feasible, especially because the interview can be quickly and cheaply scored to yield a large quantity of precoded data.

Epidemiological Research

If an epidemiological study is designed and adequately funded to perform face-to-face interviews with large samples of children, the SCICA is at least as practical as other interviews, because others also require experienced interviewers and require about the same time to administer. The SCICA is not specifically keyed to a nosology because we do not feel that valid nosological classifications can be made solely on the basis of any interviews with children. Like the SCICA, other interviews must be accompanied by additional assessment procedures as a basis for diagnosis.

Rather than interviewing all subjects in an epidemiological sample, a more economical approach is via multistage assessments. In this approach, relatively quick and inexpensive screening procedures are initially used to assess large samples. Based on the results of the initial screen, subsamples of subjects are selected for interviews. Typically, the subsamples consist of subjects who scored in the clinical range in the initial screening procedure, plus subjects selected randomly from those scoring in the normal range. Subsamples of subjects initially scoring in the normal range are selected for intensive assessment in order to determine the proportion of clinically deviant cases that would be missed by using only the initial screening procedure, i. e., the proportion of "false negatives" in the initial screening.

As examples of the multistage epidemiological strategy, studies in Holland and Puerto Rico have used translations of the CBCL and TRF to screen large general population samples (Bird et al., 1988; Verhulst, Akkerhuis, & Althaus, 1985). Subsamples of subjects scoring in the normal and clinical range were then selected for intensive evaluations that included clinical interviews. In a more specialized application of the multistage strategy, foreign children who had been adopted by Dutch parents were initially screened with the CBCL (Verhulst, Versluis-den Bieman, van der Ende, Berden, & Sanders-Woudstra, 1990). Subsamples scoring in the normal and clinical range were then assessed with clinical interviews. Although these studies were carried out before the SCICA was available, the SCICA is currently being used in similar research.

Etiological Research

The SCICA can be used in research on the etiologies of particular kinds of problems. This can be done by grouping children according to their scale scores or profile patterns on the SCICA and then comparing groups who differ on the SCICA to determine whether they differ in hypothesized etiological factors.

The reverse strategy can also be used, whereby children are grouped according to known or hypothesized differences in etiology. Children grouped by etiology can then be compared on the SCICA to determine whether the etiological factors result in differences that are detectible in the interview. Multiple measures should, of course, be used. If the SCICA and other measures failed to discriminate among children who differed in the hypothesized etiological factors, this would suggest that the hypotheses about etiology are incorrect or that assumptions about the detectible manifestations of the etiological differences are incorrect.

A third approach is to use the SCICA as a dependent variable when hypothesized etiological factors are manipulated. As an example, if it is hypothesized that particular kinds of problems can be prevented by a particular kind of intervention, a high risk group can be assigned to receive the intervention while a similar group serves as a control by receiving a different intervention or no intervention. If the group receiving the preventive intervention scores significantly lower on the target problems assessed with the SCICA, this would support the hypothesis about the etiological factors.

Outcome Studies

If we could be certain of the outcome of each child's problems under the various possible conditions of intervention or nonintervention, we would be better able to decide which children need professional help, what kind of help they need, and how to advise parents. We would also be able to concentrate research on disorders found to have poor outcomes, instead of those that are more benign.

The SCICA can be used as an outcome measure in diverse studies. For example, if we wish to know which types of children in a particular caseload typically have good versus poor outcomes, we can divide cases according to intake variables that are hypothesized to predict outcome. We can then administer the SCICA (and other standardized assessment procedures) at intake and again after a suitable follow-up interval. Children who show the most improvement from intake to follow-up can be compared with those who show the least improvement to determine what predictor variables discriminate between them. Improvement can be measured according to scores on individual SCICA items, syndromes, Internalizing, Externalizing, and/or total Observation and total Self-Report scores.

Experimental Intervention Studies

Outcome studies of the sort described in the previous section can identify groups of children who typically have good versus poor outcomes. If certain variables assessed at intake are found to predict poor outcomes with reasonable accuracy, it is important to determine how to improve outcomes for such children. This may entail trying to improve the match between the needs of these children and the available interventions or trying to develop new interventions targeted specifically on their needs. In either case, the strongest test of the efficacy of the interventions would be via an experimental design in which children in one condition receive the intervention, while children in another condition receive a different intervention or no intervention.

If the intervention is one that can be alternately activated and deactivated—such as drug treatments and certain behavioral manipulations—the same children may receive both conditions in alternating order, according to a *crossover design*. On the other hand, if the intervention cannot be switched on and off, the different treatment conditions can be assigned to groups that are selected to be similar in all other important respects. One way to attain similarity between the intervention and control groups is by randomizing assignment to treatment across the entire pool of available subjects. Greater similarity can often be achieved by creating pairs of well-matched subjects and then randomly assigning one member of each pair to each condition in a *randomized blocks design.*

Whatever experimental design is chosen, the SCICA can be used as one of the initial criteria for selecting subjects who manifest the type of problems to be treated. If a randomized blocks design is used, the SCICA scale scores can be used as one basis for creating matched pairs (or "blocks") of subjects who will then be randomly assigned to the different treatment conditions. The initial SCICA scores also provide a baseline assessment with which outcomes can be compared by readministering the SCICA after treatment.

Identifying Correlates of Disorders and Stressful Experiences

It is important to determine whether certain disorders are typically associated with other problems that may not themselves be inherent in the disorders. Medical conditions such as diabetes or asthma, for example, may often be associated with behavioral/emotional problems, which must be considered in managing the medical conditions. Changes in such problems may indicate how well the management program is working. Behavioral/emotional problems are also likely to be associated with stressful experiences, such as child abuse or the loss of a parent.

To identify problems that are associated with particular disorders or stressful experiences, the SCICA can be used to compare children who have the target condition with those who do not. It can then be determined whether children having the target condition manifest higher rates of problems overall or of particular kinds of problems. By using the SCICA and other instruments to compare children who differ with respect to particular target conditions, such as diabetes versus asthma or abuse versus loss of a parent, it can also be determined whether certain problems are specific to such conditions or whether such conditions constitute a nonspecific risk factor for increased behavioral/emotional problems in general.

APPLICATIONS TO TRAINING

Interviews are probably the most universal clinical assessment procedures. Yet, there is little uniformity in the way interviews are conducted, how interpretations are made, or how results are reported. There is still less uniformity in training people to do clinical interviews with children. In fact, training often consists of little more than observing a few interviews. Because the observed interviews are unlikely to represent much diversity of cases or techniques, the didactic base is quite meager for learning the complex skills involved in interviewing disturbed children.

In contrast to traditional interview training, the SCICA provides a standard protocol for thorough yet natural and flexible interviewing geared to children's abilities and interaction styles. It also provides standardized scoring of a large number of problems that are potentially assessable in the interview without overburdening the interviewer. Furthermore, the results are displayed in a profile format that shows where the child's problems are concentrated in comparison to other interviewees.

To facilitate training in use of the SCICA, we offer videotaped excerpts of interviews, plus scores and profiles averaged across experienced clinicians' ratings of these excerpts. Trainees can thus view and score diverse interview behaviors and compare their scores with an expert standard. If the trainees' scores differ much from those of the experienced raters, the trainees can study the taped interviews until they are able to approximate the experts' scores.

The SCICA can also be used for training by having trainees view SCICAs conducted by their clinical instructors. SCICA profiles scored by the instructor and trainee can then be compared to identify discrepancies. If the instructor's interviews are videotaped, trainees can watch them as much as necessary to improve their scoring skills. After trainees have seen and scored several interviews, they can conduct their own SCICA interviews under supervision. Trainees can benefit greatly from watching videotapes of the SCICAs that they conduct themselves.

The SCICA is intended to provide trainees not only with a particular format for conducting and scoring interviews, but also with broader concepts of clinical assessment focused on the integration of multisource data. Training should therefore include experience in systematically comparing data obtained from the interview with data obtained from other sources, such as parents, teachers, direct observations, medical examinations, and tests.

CONFIDENTIALITY

Chapter 3 outlined ways in which confidentiality issues should be discussed with interviewees. In all applications of the SCICA, it is important to protect the confidentiality of the interviewee's self-reports and other information obtained in the interview. This means that the completed SCICA Protocol, Observation and Self-Report Forms, and Profile should not be accessible to unauthorized people. For example, because school records are often accessible to many people, such as pupils who work in the school office, SCICA data should not be placed in such records.

When the SCICA is used as a basis for evaluation reports, the SCICA data should have the same confidential status as other highly personal data included in such reports. It is generally preferable to present conclusions based on multiple sources of data rather than specific statements by the interviewee or specific item scores.

SUMMARY

The SCICA is designed for clinical assessment, research, training, and the integration of each of these endeavors with the others. The SCICA is viewed as one form of direct assessment that should be used in conjunction with data from other sources, such as parents, teachers, cognitive tests, physical assessment, and observations in other settings, such as school.

Clinical applications were outlined for mental health contexts, where the SCICA can be routinely used as the initial assessment interview; school contexts, where it can be used in assessments leading to regular education interventions and in determining eligibility for special education; and forensic contexts, where it can be used in initial assessments and subsequent reassessments for custody and placement decisions and following stressful experiences, such as abuse and family disruption.

Research applications were outlined for epidemiological research; etiological research; outcome studies; experimental intervention studies; and efforts to identify the correlates of disorders and stressful experiences.

In applications to training, the SCICA provides a standard protocol for learning to interview in ways that are specifically geared to ages 6-18 and for learning to score interviews in a well-differentiated fashion. Videotaped segments of SCICA interviews are available for trainees to score and compare their scores with those of experienced raters.

Chapter 10
Case Illustrations
and Sample Report

This chapter provides case illustrations for scoring and interpreting the SCICA Profile and integrating results with other data sources. For all cases, the SCICA was part of a comprehensive assessment including parent ratings on the CBCL, teacher ratings on the TRF, parent and teacher interviews, reviews of relevant medical and educational histories, and standardized tests of intelligence and achievement. For three cases, the DOF was used to rate classroom observations. For two cases, self-ratings were obtained on the YSR. The videotape described in Chapter 3 includes simulated interviews with some of the subjects.

Assessment data are presented according to the five axes of multiaxial empirically based assessment outlined in Chapter 1. Personal details have been altered to protect confidentiality. The first case illustrates the computer-scored versions of the SCICA, CBCL, TRF, and DOF profiles. Subsequent cases illustrate the computer-scored YSR profile. The last case is formatted as a psychological evaluation to illustrate how to report results from the SCICA, CBCL, TRF, and YSR according to the multiaxial model.

PATTY, AGE 6

Patty was brought to a mental health clinic by her mother because of behavior problems at home and school. Patty's mother complained of aggressive and oppositional behavior at home, while her teacher reported hyperactivity and learning problems at school.

Axis I. Parent Reports

Patty's mother completed the CBCL and a standard background form as part of the clinic intake procedure. She was also interviewed by the psychologist who evaluated Patty.   Patty was the youngest of three children whose parents were divorced. Her mother was an unemployed high school graduate who retained custody of the three children.

On the CBCL, Patty's total competence score fell in the clinical range, while her score on the Social scale fell at the borderline clinical cutpoint. Her scores on the Activities and School scales fell in the low normal range.

Figure 10-1 shows Patty's scores on the problem scales of the computer-scored CBCL Profile. Her scores were in the clinical range on the CBCL Attention Problems, Delinquent Behavior, and Aggressive Behavior syndromes and in the borderline clinical range on the Withdrawn syndrome.   She obtained Externalizing and total problem scores in the clinical range, but her Internalizing score was in the normal range.

In addition to item scores and T scores, the computer-scored version of the CBCL prints intraclass correlations (ICCs) that indicate the degree to which the overall pattern of scores on the eight CBCL syndromes resembles profile patterns that have been identified through cluster analysis (Achenbach, 1993). An ICC of .629 indicated that Patty's overall pattern of problems on the CBCL was most similar to the Delinquent-Aggressive profile type.

Axis II. Teacher Reports

On the TRF completed by her first grade teacher, Patty's scores for total adaptive functioning and academic performance were in the borderline to clinical range. Figure 10-2 shows Patty's scores on the problem scales of the computer-scored version of the TRF Profile.

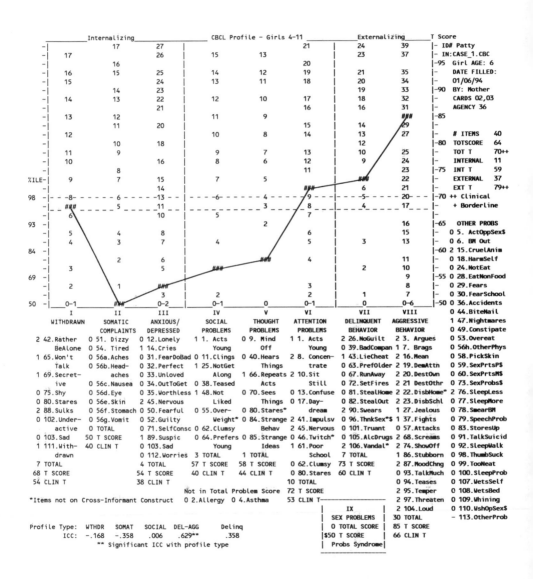

Figure 10-1. Computer-scored version of the CBCL problem scales for 6-year-old Patty.

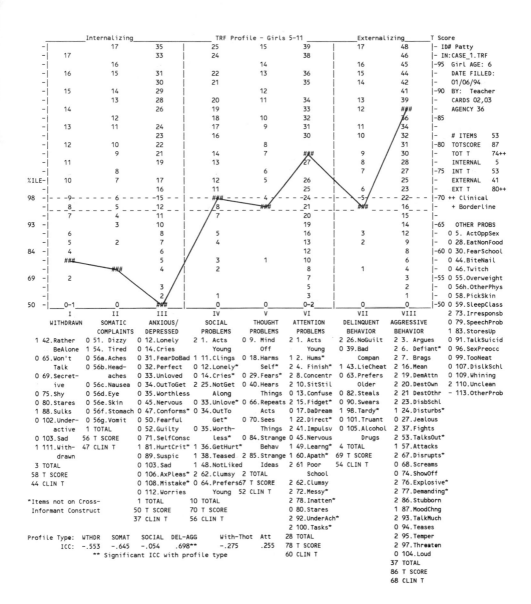

Figure 10-2. Computer-scored version of the TRF problem scales for 6-year-old Patty.

Patty's scores for Attention Problems and Aggressive Behavior were in the clinical range, while her scores for Social Problems, Thought Problems, and Delinquent Behavior were in the borderline clinical range. On the Attention Problems and Aggressive Behavior syndromes, Patty's teacher reported many problems similar to those reported by her mother on the CBCL. On the Social Problems syndrome, Patty's teacher reported such problems as acts young; clings; doesn't get along with other children; gets hurt; gets teased; not liked by other children; and clumsy. She also reported strange ideas on the Thought Problems syndrome, and lacks guilt, lies or cheats, and tardy on the Delinquent Behavior syndrome. Patty's scores on the remaining three TRF syndromes were in the normal range. Her TRF total problem and Externalizing scores were in the clinical range, while her Internalizing score was in the normal range, similar to the CBCL. As with the CBCL, Patty's overall pattern of problems on the TRF was similar to the Delinquent-Aggressive profile type (ICC = .698).

Axis III. Cognitive Assessment

On the WISC-III, Patty's scores were average to above average in all areas (FSIQ = 102), indicating no specific cognitive weaknesses. Achievement testing also showed average performance in all basic academic skills.

Axis IV. Physical Assessment

Medical records showed no evidence of physical problems. Patty's mother reported normal developmental milestones, but indicated that she had always been very active at home and difficult to discipline.

Axis V. Direct Assessment

A child psychologist at the clinic administered the SCICA. Patty was very active throughout the interview, requiring use of play materials to keep her engaged toward the end of the interview. Although Patty responded well to open-ended questions, she was resistant and often needed coaxing during the SCICA drawing tasks and achievement testing. During play activities, the psychologist incorporated questions from SCICA topic areas that were not covered by more direct questioning.

Figure 10-3 shows Patty's scores on the computer-scored SCICA Profile. Patty's total score on the SCICA Observation Form was 99, with a corresponding T score of 71, while her total score on the Self-Report Form was 46, with a corresponding T score of 59. Her Internalizing score of 14 had a T score of 49, while her Externalizing score of 101 had a T score of 81. Patty's scores for total Observations and Externalizing were above the 93rd percentile for the SCICA referred sample.

Patty's pattern of externalizing problems on the SCICA Profile is shown by T scores ranging from 68 to 79 on the Aggressive Behavior, Attention Problems, Strange, and Resistant syndromes. Scores on all four syndromes exceeded the 93rd percentile for the referred sample, as can be read from the left side of the profile. As can be seen by the items that were scored for these syndromes, Patty displayed many externalizing problems during the SCICA and reported much aggressive behavior. Patty's T score of 62 on the Family Problems syndrome was above the 80th percentile as well, but her T scores on the remaining three SCICA scales were considerably lower (T = 43 to 55).

Patty's Externalizing and total Observation scores were more than one standard deviation above the mean scores listed in Appendix C for referred and nonreferred children, as were her scores on five SCICA syndromes. Patty's scores

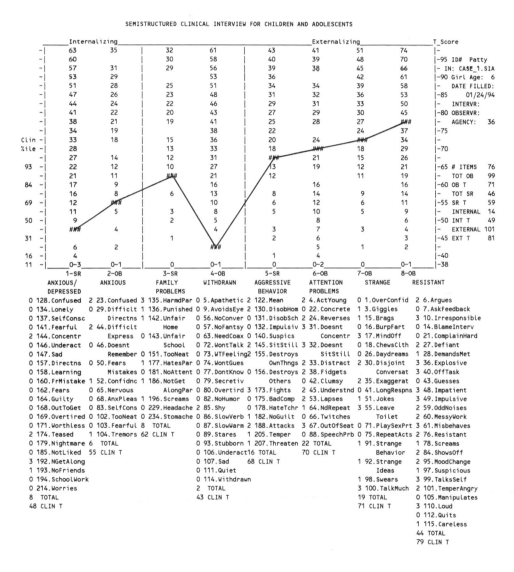

Figure 10-3. Computer-scored version of the SCICA Profile for 6-year-old Patty.

for Internalizing and the remaining three SCICA syndromes were near the mean scores for nonreferred children.

As part of the direct assessment, three 10-minute samples of Patty's behavior in school were observed and rated on the DOF, along with three samples of the behavior of two "control" girls in her class. The DOF computer program averaged the two control girls' scores for comparison with Patty's scores. Patty was on-task only 35% of the time, in contrast to an average of 95% for the control girls. Her DOF total problem, Internalizing, and Externalizing scores were in the clinical range, whereas the control girls scored in the normal range.

Figure 10-4 shows Patty's scores (solid line) on the DOF syndromes compared to the averaged scores for the control girls (broken line). Patty scored in the clinical range on the DOF Hyperactive, Attention Demanding, and Aggressive syndromes. The means of the DOF scores for the two control girls were in the normal range on all syndromes.

Summary of Findings for Patty

Patty's case illustrates consistency in severe externalizing problems reported by different informants. The SCICA Profile reflected the interviewer's observations of many externalizing problems, including attention problems along with resistant and strange behavior. The SCICA Profile also reflected Patty's reports of aggressive behavior and family problems. Patty's mother and teacher reported similar problems of an externalizing nature, including aggressive behavior and attention problems, plus violations of social rules. Patty's teacher also reported social problems. Direct observations in Patty's classroom corroborated the teacher's report and revealed more externalizing problems than shown by two randomly selected girls in the same classroom. Scores on all four empirically based measures thus showed considerably more problems than are typically reported for girls of Patty's age. Despite these behavior problems, Patty

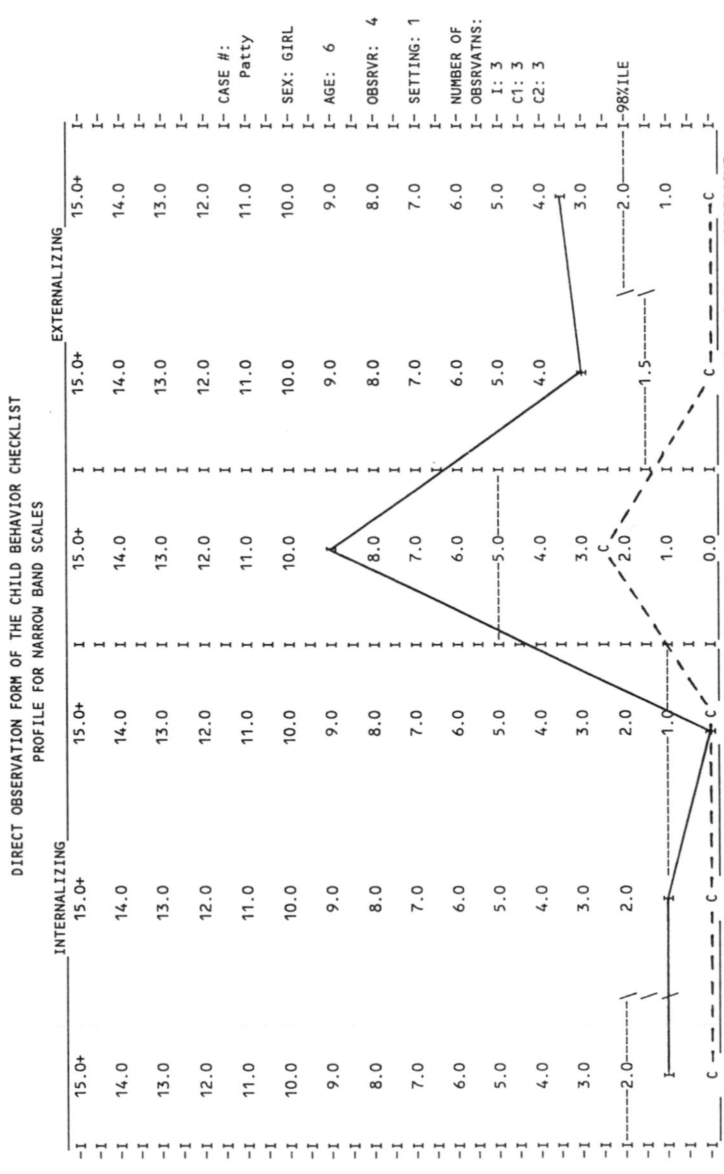

Figure 10-4. Computer-scored version of the DOF syndrome scales for 6-year-old Patty. (Item scores omitted.)

obtained scores in the average range on the WISC-III and achievement tests. The results of the comprehensive assessment led to behavioral interventions at home and school, combined with stimulant medication pursuant to a DSM-IV diagnosis of Attention Deficit Hyperactivity Disorder (ADHD). A diagnosis of Oppositional Defiant Disorder (ODD) was also appropriate.

BRUCE, AGE 9

Bruce was referred to a psychiatric outpatient clinic for evaluation of his cognitive and social-emotional functioning. Bruce's parents expressed concerns about social withdrawal at home and restless, inattentive behavior. They also reported that his school performance was erratic and that his teacher told them he displayed "odd" social behaviors.

Axis I. Parent Reports

Bruce was brought to the clinic by his mother, who provided background information. Bruce was the middle child in a blended family of three children. His parents divorced when Bruce was 2 years old. Bruce's mother, who retained custody of the children, remarried 2 years later. Bruce's biological father was placed in a state hospital, diagnosed as having a major mental disorder, after which the children did not communicate with him. In his early years, Bruce was socially withdrawn and delayed in speech and motor development. He also exhibited self-stimulatory behavior, such as rubbing his stomach, rocking, and hitting himself. A psychological evaluation at age 4 indicated cognitive ability in the mildly retarded range and mentioned "autistic-like" behavior. Based on this evaluation, Bruce began receiving special education services at school.

Bruce's mother completed the CBCL as part of the intake procedure for his evaluation at age 9. Bruce's CBCL total competence score fell in the normal range, as did his scores on the Activities and Social scales. His score on the School scale fell in the borderline clinical range.

Bruce's CBCL total problem score fell in the clinical range, while his Internalizing score fell in the borderline clinical range. His Externalizing score was well within the normal range. On the CBCL syndromes, Bruce scored in the clinical range for Social Problems and Attention Problems, and in the borderline clinical range for Thought Problems. Bruce's mother endorsed 7 of 8 possible items on the Social Problems syndrome, including acts young and prefers younger children, along with other items indicating poor peer relations. She endorsed all 11 items on the Attention Problems syndrome, scoring 8 of the items 2, including can't concentrate; can't sit still; confused; daydreams; impulsive; nervous; twitches; and clumsy. On the Thought Problems syndrome, Bruce's mother endorsed obsessive thoughts; repetitive actions; and stares blankly. Bruce's scores on all other CBCL syndromes fell in the normal range. An ICC of .590 indicated that Bruce's overall pattern of problems was most similar to the Social Problems profile type.

Axis II. Teacher Reports

Bruce attended a regular third grade classroom, but also received speech and language services. His teacher rated his adaptive functioning on the TRF in the clinical range, but she rated his academic performance as above average in math and average in all other subjects.

Bruce's TRF total problem score fell in the clinical range, while his Externalizing score fell in the borderline clinical range. His scores were in the borderline to clinical range on the TRF Social Problems, Thought Problems, and Attention Problems syndromes, based on problems similar to those reported by his mother on the CBCL. In addition, Bruce's teacher gave ratings of 2 for TRF items *84. Strange behavior* and *85. Strange ideas*, describing bizarre acts and disjointed, illogical thoughts. Bruce's scores on the remaining five TRF scales fell in the normal range, although his teacher did score 14 items on the Aggressive Behavior syndrome, yielding a score above the 80th percentile.

Axis III. Cognitive Assessment

The WISC-III yielded a Full Scale IQ of 94, but a large discrepancy between Bruce's verbal score (VIQ = 112) and performance score (PIQ = 77). Bruce showed strengths in verbal reasoning and acquired knowledge, but weaknesses in visual-spatial reasoning. During the WISC-III, Bruce had particular difficulty recognizing and reproducing puzzle patterns. Although he answered verbal items appropriately, he often strayed from the original topic, and his thoughts seemed disorganized. Nonetheless, Bruce's scores on the WISC-III verbal comprehension and distractibility factors were in the average range. The Bender Visual Motor Gestalt Test also showed below average visual-motor integration, with a Koppitz (1975) age equivalent of 6 years. Achievement testing indicated above average performance in math and average performance in other basic academic skills.

Axis IV. Physical Assessment

Bruce's medical history showed no serious illnesses or physical problems other than developmental delays reported by his mother. A neurological exam at age 4 had identified problems in attention and eye-hand coordination, along with delays in fine and gross motor skills. At age 9, no medical or physical problems were evident.

Axis V. Direct Assessment

The SCICA was administered by a child psychiatrist at the outpatient clinic. Although Bruce was friendly and cooperative during the interview, he avoided eye contact and seemed socially immature and awkward. He had difficulty expressing this thoughts, resulting in loose and disjointed conversation. His thinking seemed overly concrete when he described physical details of objects or people and demonstrated his ideas through actions. Bruce also seemed preoccupied with certain thoughts, especially his interest in football, which often intruded into other topics. Bruce expressed a positive attitude toward school, and seemed particularly knowledgeable about math and science. His conversation about his family centered on activities more than relationships, except for arguments with his mother and siblings. He reported having no close friends and was very concerned about being teased and picked on by his peers.

Figure 10-5 displays Bruce's scores on the computer-scored SCICA profile. Bruce's T scores for total Observations, total Self-Reports, Internalizing, and Externalizing ranged from 47 to 58, which were near the 50th percentile for referred children. The SCICA profile showed peaks for observed problems on the Anxious and Strange syndromes, with T scores exceeding the 90th percentile for referred children. Bruce's T score on the Attention Problems syndrome exceeded the 80th percentile. Bruce also reported several social problems that are scored on the Anxious/-Depressed syndrome, as well as other problems scored on the Aggressive Behavior syndrome. In contrast to other syndromes, very few items were scored on the Resistant syndrome.

Bruce's score on the SCICA Strange syndrome was more than one standard deviation above the mean for referred children, while his score on the Resistant syndrome was one standard deviation below the mean. His scores on all other SCICA scales were comparable to the mean scores for referred children. Bruce's scores on 8 of the 12 SCICA scales were more than one standard deviation above mean scores for nonreferred children.

The SCICA T scores can also be compared to clinical T scores obtained on comparable scales of the CBCL and

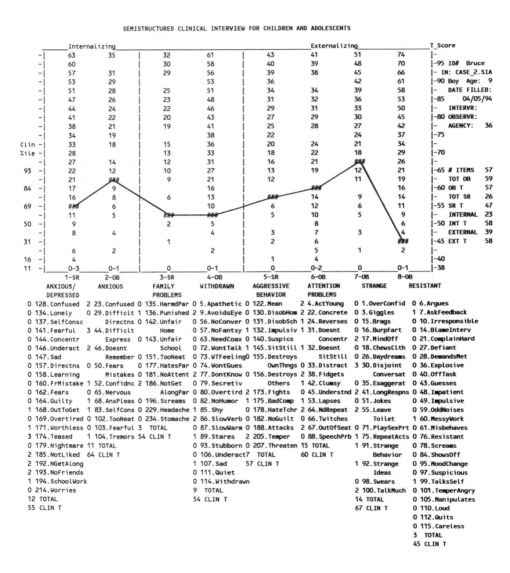

Figure 10-5. Computer-scored version of the SCICA Profile for 9-year-old Bruce.

TRF. The clinical *T* scores, printed on the computer-scored CBCL and TRF, indicate how an individual's scale scores compare to scores of a clinically referred sample. Bruce's *T* score of 67 on the SCICA Strange syndrome was similar to his clinical *T* score of 67 on the TRF Thought Problems syndrome, and higher than his clinical *T* score of 53 on CBCL Thought Problems. His *T* score of 60 on the SCICA Attention Problems syndrome was similar to his clinical *T* score of 55 on TRF Attention Problems, and lower than his clinical *T* score of 92 on CBCL Attention Problems.

A special education aide rated Bruce's school behavior on the DOF on three occasions in his third grade classroom. He was on-task only 45% of the time, compared to an average of 90% for two control boys. His DOF total problem score was in the clinical range and much higher than the average of two control boys. His DOF Internalizing score was also in the clinical range, whereas his Externalizing score was in the normal range. Unlike the control boys, Bruce's scores on the DOF Withdrawn-Inattentive and Hyperactive syndromes were in the clinical range, and his score on the Nervous-Obsessive syndrome fell just at the clinical cutpoint. The observer scored such problems as can't concentrate; can't sit still; fidgets; bites nails; easily distracted; talks too much; stares blankly; and nervous movements. On the playground, Bruce screamed constantly, made odd sounds, and seemed overly anxious to please other children in games.

Summary of Findings for Bruce

Bruce's case illustrates consistency across data sources in ratings of strange behavior, thought problems, and social problems. The cross-informant computer program for the CBCL and TRF indicated above average agreement between ratings by Bruce's mother and his teacher, including borderline to clinical range scores on the Social Problems, Thought Problems, and Attention Problems syndromes. An elevated score on the SCICA Strange syndrome was consistent with high scores on the CBCL and TRF Thought Problems syndromes. A high score on the SCICA Anxious syndrome also reflected confusion, difficulty expressing thoughts, memory lapses, and other associated problems. Classroom observations scored on the DOF identified attention problems and hyperactivity that were consistent with results on the SCICA, CBCL, and TRF. The cognitive assessment showed further evidence of disorganized thinking that became apparent during the SCICA, along with a wide discrepancy between verbal and performance ability. However, Bruce's IQ scores had improved since he was first assessed at age 4.

The findings from the multiaxial assessment indicated similar problems across different situations, including the clinical interview and home and school environments. His father's major mental disorder was an important factor to consider in the etiology of Bruce's problems. The disruptive effects of his father's commitment to a psychiatric hospital and subsequent parental divorce may have also hindered Bruce's early cognitive and social development. The ratings obtained at age 9 showed disordered thinking, social problems, and attention problems, even after Bruce's cognitive functioning and family situation had improved. Although Bruce met many criteria for a DSM-IV diagnosis of Attention Deficit-Hyperactivity Disorder (ADHD), such a diagnosis fails to capture the unusual quality of his thought processes and his strange behavior, or the unevenness of his cognitive abilities.

Bruce continued to receive speech and language services in school. Recommendations were also made to school staff for structuring his educational environment and developing better social skills. Pharmacotherapy trials were initiated by the attending psychiatrist at the outpatient clinic to assess the efficacy of medication for Bruce's attention problems.

CATHERINE, AGE 11

Catherine was referred to a school psychologist by her teacher, because she seemed inattentive and withdrawn, was having difficulty in reading and written work, and was erratic in completing assignments. She had few friends in school and sometimes seemed very sad. An evaluation was requested to assess her emotional functioning and possible learning disabilities.

Axis I. Parent Reports

Catherine was the youngest of two children living with her mother. Her father died when she was 7 years old, and her mother had not remarried. Her mother was college educated and worked as an accountant.

Catherine's mother completed the CBCL prior to an interview with the school psychologist. Catherine's CBCL total competence score was in the borderline clinical range. Her scores on the Activities and School scales were in the borderline to clinical range, while her score on the Social scale was in the low normal range. These results indicated limited social involvement and poor school performance consistent with the teacher's referral concerns.

Catherine's CBCL total problem score fell in the borderline clinical range, while her Internalizing score fell in the clinical range. Catherine's Externalizing score was in the normal range. Her score on the CBCL Withdrawn syndrome was in the clinical range, while her scores on all other CBCL syndromes were in the normal range. Catherine's mother endorsed 8 of 9 possible items on the Withdrawn syndrome: would rather be alone; won't talk; shy or timid; stares; sulks; underactive; unhappy, sad or depressed; and withdrawn. She also reported stubbornness, mood changes, temper tantrums, and sleep problems, as well as social problems and attention problems. An ICC of .605

indicated that Catherine's overall pattern of problems on the CBCL was most similar to the Withdrawn profile type.

Axis II. Teacher Reports

The TRF completed by Catherine's fifth grade teacher yielded adaptive functioning and academic performance scores in the clinical range. Catherine's teacher rated her particularly low on how hard she was working and how much she was learning, and indicated that she was achieving far below grade level in most subjects.

Catherine's TRF total problem and Internalizing scores fell in the clinical range, while her Externalizing score fell in the normal range. Catherine's scores were in the borderline to clinical range on four TRF syndromes: Withdrawn, Anxious/Depressed, Thought Problems, and Attention Problems. On the Withdrawn syndrome, Catherine's teacher endorsed 8 of the 9 items, most of which were similar to those endorsed by her mother on the CBCL. On the Anxious/Depressed syndrome, the teacher endorsed such problems as feels worthless; feels guilty; self conscious; feels hurt when criticized; unhappy, sad or depressed; and overly anxious to please. The teacher endorsed 16 of the 20 items on the Attention Problems syndrome, including fails to finish things; can't concentrate; confused; daydreaming; poor school work; and other attentional and organizational problems. The teacher also scored obsessions and strange behavior on the Thought Problems syndrome. Scores on the remaining four TRF syndromes were in the normal range, although Catherine's teacher did report social problems and mood changes. Catherine's overall pattern of problems on the TRF was most similar to the Withdrawn profile type (ICC = .734), as was also found on the CBCL.

Axis III. Cognitive Assessment

Catherine cooperated well during cognitive and achievement testing and appeared to enjoy the attention. She seemed to lack confidence, responded slowly when unsure of her answers, and needed frequent coaxing. She performed best on visual tasks, showing good discrimination and spatial reasoning. Her slow reading accelerated in response to praise.

The WISC-III revealed superior ability (FSIQ = 125), with no signs of cognitive deficits. Achievement testing yielded average scores for fifth grade in all basic academic skills, including reading and writing. Though Catherine's IQ scores would predict higher achievement, there was no evidence of learning disabilities.

Axis IV. Physical Assessment

Catherine was of normal height and weight. Medical records showed some complications at birth and problems with colic as an infant. She was prone to ear infections and had frequent somatic complaints during her early development. Developmental milestones were normal, but Catherine had always seemed moody as a child, according to her mother. No further medical examination seemed warranted.

Axis V. Direct Assessment

The school psychologist asked Catherine to complete the YSR prior to administering the SCICA. The school psychologist also observed and rated Catherine's behavior in the classroom, using the DOF.

Catherine's self-ratings on the YSR produced a total competence score within the normal range. Figure 10-6 shows Catherine's scores on the problem scales of the computer-scored YSR. Her total problem and Internalizing scores were in the clinical range, while her Externalizing

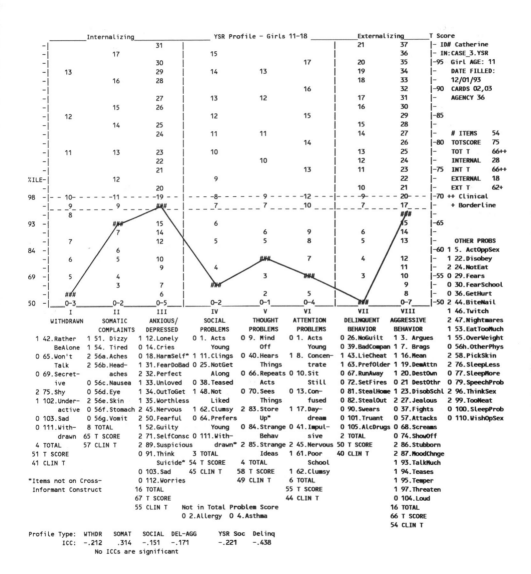

Figure 10-6. Computer-scored version of the YSR problem scales for 11-year-old Catherine.

score was in the borderline clinical range. Catherine scored in the borderline clinical range on the YSR Anxious/ Depressed syndrome, and just below the borderline clinical range on the Aggressive Behavior syndrome. Items endorsed by Catherine on the Anxious/Depressed syndrome were consistent with problems reported by her teacher on the TRF, with the exception of a score of *0* for YSR item *103. Unhappy, sad, or depressed*, which had been scored *1* by her teacher and *2* by her mother. Catherine endorsed more items than her teacher or her mother on the Aggressive Behavior syndrome, including argues; brags; mean; jealous; stubborn; mood changes; and temper tantrums, but no problems reflecting physical aggression. Low ICCs on the YSR indicated that the overall pattern of problems reported by Catherine did not match any specific profile type.

During the SCICA, Catherine appeared sad, withdrawn, and anxious much of the time. Her self-reports revealed unresolved grief about the death of her father. She acknowledged that she still missed her father and thought about him a lot, even during school hours. She was somewhat reluctant to discuss her sad feelings and said she did not talk about them with her mother or anyone else, such as a counselor.

Figure 10-7 shows Catherine's scores on the SCICA profile. Her Internalizing *T* score of 65 was above the 93rd percentile for referred children, while her Externalizing *T* score of 42 was at about the 20th percentile. Her scores for total Observations and total Self-Reports were around the 70th percentile for referred children. The SCICA profile showed peaks on the Anxious and Withdrawn syndromes, with scores ≥93rd percentile. The interviewer endorsed 10 of the 12 items on the Anxious syndrome and 15 of the 21 items on the Withdrawn syndrome. Catherine's self-reported problems on the Anxious/Depressed syndrome included being lonely; being fearful; unhappy, sad, or depressed; fears; being overtired; getting teased; nightmares; not liked; problems getting along with other children;

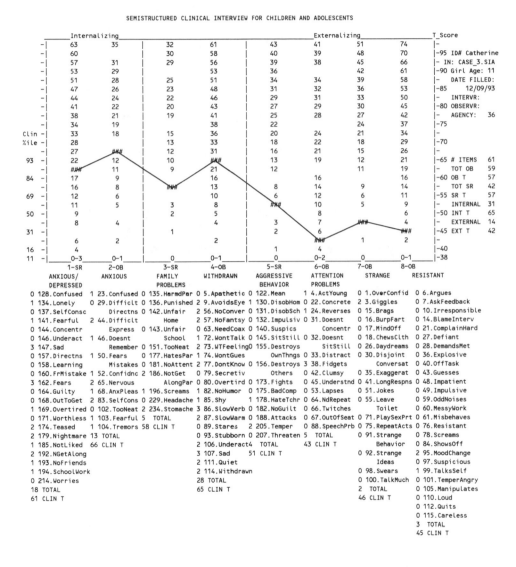

Figure 10-7. Computer-scored SCICA Profile for 11-year-old Catherine.

problems making friends; and problems with school work. On the Family Problems syndrome, Catherine reported not getting along with her mother; screaming; and stomachaches. Very few items were scored on the SCICA externalizing syndromes.

Catherine's total Self-Report and Internalizing scores on the SCICA were more than one standard deviation above the mean for referred children. Her Externalizing score was one standard deviation below the mean. Catherine's scores on the SCICA Anxious and Withdrawn syndromes were also more than one standard deviation above the mean scores for referred children, indicating severe problems in these areas. Her scores on the four SCICA externalizing syndromes were far below those of referred children and similar to the mean scores for nonreferred children, indicating very few externalizing problems. Catherine's T score of 65 on the SCICA Withdrawn syndrome was similar to her clinical T scores on the Withdrawn syndrome of the CBCL (67) and TRF (63). Catherine's T score of 66 on the SCICA Anxious syndrome was similar to her clinical T scores on the Anxious/Depressed syndromes of the TRF (61) and YSR (67).

Classroom observations scored on the DOF indicated that Catherine was on-task only 45% of the time, compared to an average of 85% for two control girls in the same classroom. Catherine's total problem score on the DOF was in the clinical range and higher than the average score of the other two girls. Her Internalizing score was also in the clinical range, whereas her Externalizing score was in the normal range. On the DOF Withdrawn-Inattentive and Hyperactive syndromes, Catherine scored much higher than the control girls and well into the clinical range. Observed problems included can't concentrate; can't sit still; daydreaming; staring; fidgets; easily distracted; nail biting; and talks too much. During recess, Catherine spent most of her time standing alone watching other children.

Summary of Findings for Catherine

Catherine's case illustrates general consistency among different informants in their reports of severe internalizing problems, consisting of withdrawal, anxiety, and depression. However, there were some differences between problems reported by Catherine and those reported by her mother and teacher. The cross-informant computer program indicated above average agreement between ratings by Catherine's mother on the CBCL and her teacher on the TRF. There was average agreement between Catherine's self ratings on the YSR and ratings by her teacher, but below average agreement between Catherine and her mother. On the YSR, Catherine reported many problems on the Anxious/Depressed syndrome, but fewer problems on the Withdrawn syndrome.

The SCICA revealed problems similar to those reported by both Catherine's mother and teacher, as well as by Catherine herself on the YSR. The elevated score on the SCICA Withdrawn syndrome was similar to clinical T scores on the CBCL and TRF Withdrawn syndromes, while her elevated score on the SCICA Anxious syndrome was similar to clinical T scores on the TRF and YSR Anxious/Depressed syndromes. The SCICA further revealed Catherine's unresolved sadness about the death of her father, although she did not score herself as being unhappy on the YSR. Classroom observations with the DOF further corroborated the teacher's report of withdrawal and attention problems.

The cognitive assessment by the school psychologist showed superior ability and no cognitive deficits, indicating that Catherine's academic problems were more likely due to emotional problems than to learning disabilities. Based on results of the multiaxial assessment, Catherine met criteria for the special education disability category of Serious Emotional Disturbance (SED), as discussed in Chapter 9. Catherine remained in her fifth grade classroom, but an Individualized Education Program (IEP) was developed to reduce social withdrawal, improve social skills, and provide academic support for organizing and completing assignments.

The pattern of Catherine's problems met criteria for a DSM-IV diagnosis of Dysthymia. Information from Catherine's mother was used to judge onset and duration criteria relevant to Dysthymia. Catherine was referred to a mental health clinic for individual and family therapy.

KARL, AGE 12

Karl's case is presented in the format of a psychological evaluation report to illustrate how users can present results from the SCICA in conjunction with the CBCL, TRF, and YSR.

Psychological Evaluation

Name: Karl Bryant, Jr.
Date of Birth: 1/10/82
Chronological Age: 12 years, 1 month
Grade: Sixth
Date of Evaluation: 2/17/94

Reason for Referral

Karl was referred for a psychoeducational evaluation by his school's Basic Staffing Team (BST). Karl's sixth grade teacher reported aggressive behavior, poor peer relations, and frequent violation of school rules. Karl also failed to complete assignments, resulting in failing grades in several subjects. The psychological evaluation was requested as part of a comprehensive assessment to determine whether Karl needed special education services. Karl's mother also wanted advice on how to manage his behavior at home.

Assessment Procedures

Child Behavior Checklist (CBCL)
Teacher's Report Form (TRF)
Wechsler Intelligence Scale for Children-Third Edition
  (WISC-III)
Semistructured Clinical Interview for Children and
  Adolescents (SCICA)
Youth Self-Report (YSR)
Parent and Teacher Interviews
Record Review

Parent Reports

Karl's mother, Nancy Ladd, reported that he was the oldest in a blended family of two children. Karl's biological parents were divorced when he was 5 years old and both have remarried. Karl lives with his mother, who has custody, his stepfather (Robert Ladd), and one stepsister (Casey, age 7). Mrs. Ladd holds a 2-year college degree and works as a legal secretary. Mr. Ladd works as a plant manager in a local manufacturing company.

Karl's biological father (Karl Bryant, Sr.) lives in a different state. He has held several jobs, and currently works in a retail store. Karl visits his father over Christmas vacation and for the entire month of July. Karl's mother reported that Mr. Bryant was alcoholic, as was his own father, and that he was violent and abusive toward herself and Karl prior to the divorce. She also reported she had problems with depression during the divorce period and that her own mother suffered from depression. Mrs. Ladd reported normal developmental milestones for Karl, but a history of behavior problems since he was 4 years old, including hyperactivity, a quick temper, and resistance to discipline. She said he continues to show similar problems, although now seems less "hyper." She felt that his behavior problems increased after visits with his father.

Karl's mother completed the *Child Behavior Checklist* (CBCL) to provide her perceptions of his competencies and problems over the past 6 months. Karl's total competence score fell in the clinical range (below 10th percentile) for boys aged 12-18. He scored in the borderline clinical range on the Social and School scales. Karl's score on the Activities scale was in the normal range. Karl's mother indicated that he belongs to no social organizations and has only one friend whom he sees 1-2 times per week. She rated his school performance as failing in three subjects and below average in two subjects. She indicated that he has not repeated any grades and is not in a special class, but that he has had problems in school since first grade.

On the CBCL problem scales, Karl scored in the clinical range (above 90th percentile) for total problems and Externalizing, and in the borderline clinical range for Internalizing. Karl scored in the borderline to clinical range (≥95th percentile) on the Thought Problems, Aggressive Behavior, and Delinquent Behavior syndromes. He scored near the borderline clinical range on the Anxious/Depressed, Social Problems, and Attention Problems syndromes. On the Thought Problems syndrome, Karl's mother reported that he can't get his mind off certain thoughts, repeats certain acts over and over, and sometimes exhibits strange behavior and strange ideas. On the Delinquent Behavior and Aggressive Behavior syndromes, Karl's mother reported such problems as: lacks guilt; hangs around kids who get in trouble; lies or cheats; steals at home and elsewhere; swears; argues; mean to other children; disobeys at home and school; fights; physically attacks others; mood changes; stubborn; and temper tantrums.

Teacher Reports

Karl's sixth grade teacher reported several in-school detentions for aggressive and defiant behavior and one suspension for smoking on school grounds. The teacher reported that several behavior management approaches have been tried with Karl. At the time of evaluation, Karl was on a point system to help him complete his work and behave appropriately in class. He occasionally met with the school guidance counselor, but was not receiving any other special services.

On the *Teacher's Report Form* (TRF), Karl's teacher rated his academic performance as failing in three subjects and somewhat below grade level in two subjects, producing an academic performance score in the clinical range (below 10th percentile). Karl's total adaptive functioning score also fell in the clinical range. Compared to other students, Karl's teacher gave him low scores for working hard, behaving appropriately, learning, and happiness.

On the TRF problem scales, Karl scored in the clinical range (above the 90th percentile) for total problems, Internalizing, and Externalizing. Karl scored in the borderline to clinical range ($\geq$95th percentile) on the Anxious/Depressed, Social Problems, Delinquent Behavior, and Aggressive Behavior syndromes. He scored in the normal range on all other TRF scales, including Attention Problems. Karl's teacher endorsed 22 of 25 items on the Aggressive Behavior syndrome, including many of the same problems reported by his mother on the CBCL. On the Delinquent Behavior syndrome, Karl's teacher also reported problems similar to those reported by his mother, with the exception of lying or cheating and stealing (both scored *0*). Karl's teacher reported more problems than did his mother on the Anxious/Depressed and Social Problems syndromes. Examples included: cries; feels others are out to get him; nervous; fearful; feels hurt when criticized; suspicious; unhappy, sad, or depressed; doesn't get along with other children; gets teased; and not liked.

Cognitive Assessment

The *Wechsler Intelligence Scale for Children-III* (WISC-III) was used to measure Karl's cognitive strengths and weaknesses. Karl was friendly and engaging in conversation, but somewhat restless while answering WISC-III verbal items. He used an analytic and careful approach to WISC-III performance items. The WISC-III scores appear to be valid indices of Karl's current cognitive functioning.

Karl's Verbal IQ was in the high average range, while his Performance and Full Scale IQs were in the average range. Karl's IQ scores and Index scores on the scales of the WISC-III are listed below in terms of standard scores and percentiles. Standard scores have a mean of 100 and a standard deviation of 15.

Scale	*Score*	*Per- centile*	*95% Confi- dence Interval*
Verbal IQ	112	79	105-118
Performance IQ	102	55	94-110
Full Scale IQ	107	68	101-112
Verbal Comprehension Index	110	75	103-116
Perceptual Organization Index	105	63	96-113
Freedom from Distractibility Index	101	53	92-110
Processing Speed Index	96	39	87-106

On the verbal subtests of the WISC-III, Karl scored in the average to high average range for general information, abstract verbal reasoning, numerical reasoning, expressive vocabulary, and practical reasoning. He scored in the low average range for auditory attention span. On the performance subtests, Karl scored in the average range in all areas, including discrimination of fine detail in pictures, perceptual motor speed, visual sequencing around a social theme, abstract nonverbal reasoning, recognition of part-whole relations in familiar objects, and visual scanning. Karl's scores on the WISC-III subtests are listed below. Scores of 8 to 12 are in the average range.

Verbal		*Performance*	
Information	10	Picture Completion	12
Similarities	13	Coding	8
Arithmetic	13	Picture Arrangement	11
Vocabulary	11	Block Design	10
Comprehension	13	Object Assembly	10
Digit Span	7	Symbol Search	10

Standardized achievement tests showed low average to average scores in all areas. Details are provided in the special educator's report.

Physical Assessment

Karl is an attractive young man of normal height and weight. Medical records showed no serious medical or physical problems. At age 6, Karl was prescribed Ritalin for Attention Deficit Hyperactivity Disorder (ADHD), diagnosed by the family pediatrician. His mother reported reduced overactivity and some improvement in school grades. Medication was discontinued at age 8 after its effectiveness seemed to decrease.

Direct Assessment of Karl

Karl completed the *Youth Self-Report* (YSR) prior to being interviewed. His total competence score was well within the normal range for self-ratings by boys aged 11-18, including normal range scores on the YSR Activities and Social scales. These scores were in sharp contrast to the low competence scores on the CBCL completed by Karl's mother.

On the YSR problem scales, Karl scored in the borderline clinical range for Externalizing, but in the normal range for total problems and Internalizing. He scored in the borderline clinical range ($\geq$95th percentile) on the Withdrawn syndrome, endorsing as "very true or often true" such items as: would rather be alone; secretive; underactive; and withdrawn. Although he reported several problems on the Delinquent Behavior and Aggressive Behavior syndromes, these scale scores were somewhat below the borderline clinical range. Examples of items endorsed on these syndromes included lacks guilt; hangs around with kids who get in trouble; prefers older children; and several items describing verbal and physical aggression, which were scored *1*.

The *Semistructured Clinical Interview for Children and Adolescents* (SCICA) was administered to assess Karl's behavioral and emotional functioning in relation to school, family, friends, and personal issues. During the SCICA, Karl sometimes fidgeted with objects, but was only mildly restless and distractible. He engaged easily in conversation and seemed eager to discuss his current problems. His mood fluctuated from a happy, pleasant demeanor when discussing his interests, to intense anger when discussing problems with teachers and peers at school. Karl complained that the SCICA achievement tests were hard, and he occasionally needed to have questions repeated. Karl tended to boast about his intellectual ability, but also acknowledged problems completing school work. He also boasted about his physical strength, saying no one at school could "take him" in fights. He openly described physical fights with other students. Some of these battles were initiated by him through physical attacks seeking revenge for something he considered an insult or an injustice. He also acknowledged breaking school rules, which led to detentions. Karl was very concerned about fairness, a theme that repeatedly intruded into other topics. He complained that teachers singled him out for punishment and blamed him for things that were not his fault. Karl also described his bad temper, saying that anger builds up inside him until he loses control.

Karl expressed more positive feelings about his home situation. Though he acknowledged behavior problems at home, he felt that parental discipline was much fairer than discipline at school. He was especially enthusiastic about a point system used at home. Karl's self-reports during the SCICA suggested limited social coping strategies. For problems with peers, he mainly used physical aggression, while for problems with school authorities, he was mainly defiant. He stated that he had many friends who were often in trouble. He expressed special interest in outdoor activities that were physically challenging and risky (e.g., rock climbing, downhill skiing).

The SCICA Profile (Figure 10-8) produced total Observation and Internalizing scores that were similar to those obtained by other clinically referred children. In contrast, Karl's total Self-Report and Externalizing scores were more than one standard deviation higher than scores for referred children. Karl's scores for self-reported problems on the Aggressive Behavior syndrome and observed problems on the Strange syndrome exceeded the 93rd percentile for referred children. Because the SCICA scores provide comparisons to other referred children (not normative samples), they indicate exceptionally severe problems.

Summary of Findings

Multiple sources revealed severe behavioral and emotional problems. The CBCL from Karl's mother and the TRF from his teacher both showed severe internalizing and externalizing problems. Karl's mother and teacher agreed in their reports of severe aggressive and delinquent behavior, producing scores in the borderline to clinical range on the relevant CBCL and TRF syndromes. Karl's mother also

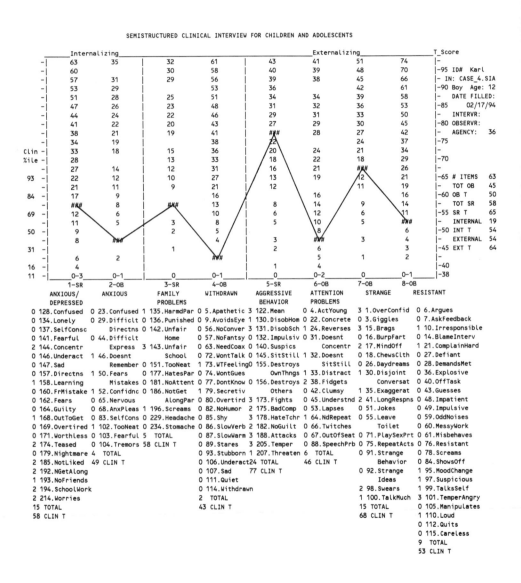

Figure 10-8. Computer-scored SCICA Profile for 12-year-old Karl.

reported thought problems, while his teacher reported anxiety, unhappiness, and social problems.

Direct assessment also indicated more severe problems than found for most boys of Karl's age. Karl's ratings of his own problems on the YSR produced borderline clinical range scores for externalizing problems and withdrawal, but lower scores on all other YSR syndromes. In a semistructured clinical interview, Karl reported aggressive behavior and social problems that were consistent with parent and teacher reports. Karl also exhibited mood changes from a pleasant demeanor when discussing his interests to intense anger when discussing problems with teachers and peers at school. He was very concerned about fairness. Although Karl expressed positive feelings about his home situation, he did acknowledge behavior problems at home as well as at school. Karl's reports during the interview suggested limited social coping strategies. His main strategy was to use physical aggression toward peers and defiance toward school authority figures.

As assessed from multiple perspectives, Karl's pattern of behavioral and emotional problems is consistent with a DSM-IV diagnosis of Conduct Disorder. His problems also meet special education criteria for Serious Emotional Disturbance (SED), as defined in the Individuals with Disabilities Education Act (IDEA). There was substantial evidence of the SED characteristic of "inappropriate types of behavior or feelings under normal circumstances." There was also evidence of "an inability to build or maintain satisfactory relationships with peers and teachers." Borderline to clinical range scores on standardized rating scales demonstrated that Karl's problems were of "a marked degree" compared to norms for boys his age. Reports by Karl's mother and school staff indicated that his problems have existed for "a long period of time." Reports by school staff also provided evidence of "adverse effects on educational performance" in terms of failing grades and frequent detentions and suspensions.

Cognitive assessment demonstrated average overall intellectual functioning and high average verbal ability. Karl showed average to high average ability on all of the WISC-III subtests, indicating no specific cognitive deficits that might interfere with his academic performance. In spite of average IQ and achievement test scores, Karl's teacher reported that he often does not complete assignments and is failing three sixth grade subjects.

Family factors are important considerations for understanding Karl's behavioral and emotional problems. Mrs. Ladd reported that Karl's biological father was alcoholic and had been violent and abusive toward herself and Karl prior to the parental divorce when Karl was age 5. Mrs. Ladd reported being depressed during the divorce period. She also reported that Karl has had behavior problems since age 4, including hyperactivity, a quick temper, and oppositional behavior. Discipline in the home has been inconsistent and has become increasingly difficult as Karl approaches adolescence.

On the positive side, Karl has an engaging and enthusiastic personality. Though he tends to be argumentative and resistant to adult authority figures, he has responded positively to behavior management programs combining rewards with clear limits and predictable consequences for infractions. It is also important to provide Karl a sense of control over alternatives in his life. A collaborative approach is recommended for addressing Karl's problems, involving mental health, home, and school interventions, as detailed below.

Recommendations

On the basis of the present evaluation, the following recommendations are offered regarding special education eligibility and behavioral/emotional problems. The special educator's report provides additional recommendations regarding academic needs.

1. Standardized rating scales and the clinical evaluation indicate that Karl meets criteria for Serious Emotional Disturbance (SED), as defined by special education law. Behavioral rating scales indicate more severe problems than are typical of boys Karl's age. Past history indicates that Karl's problems have been present for a long period of time. His failing grades and school discipline problems indicate that Karl needs special education interventions to succeed in the school setting.

2. A structured behavior management plan is recommended for reducing aggressive and oppositional behavior and for improving Karl's social and adaptive functioning at school, including the following components:

   a. Clearly defined behavioral targets, limited to 3 or 4 behaviors at any one time.

   b. A point system for promoting the behavioral goals.

   c. Clearly specified rewards and consequences.

   d. A menu of rewards, including both material and social rewards.

   e. A clear warning system and time-out procedures.

   f. Opportunities to engage in problem solving regarding future events and behavior.

3. As indicated above, both material and social rewards are important for Karl. Money is a good motivator and is developmentally appropriate for a young adolescent. Social rewards could include time with a favorite and supportive adult. Physical activities are also likely to be reinforcing, especially challenging outdoor activities.

4. Karl needs frequent and consistent praise to reinforce desirable social behavior and academic achievement. Praising small accomplishments or incremental steps in a sequence of skills would be especially helpful. Examples are praising him for completing parts of assignments, getting materials ready on time, and cooperating in group activities. Karl is very sensitive to any form of criticism. It would be helpful if teachers avoided marking his errors with red pencils. A better approach would be to note positive aspects of his work, followed by instructions for improvement.

5. Karl is prone to power struggles and oppositional behavior. He often responds negatively to adult requests. The following strategies can help to reduce noncompliance:

a. Briefly ignoring negative responses while waiting for compliance.

b. Setting time limits for compliance.

c. Using time-outs and requiring Karl to "make up the time" wasted when he refuses to comply.

d. Providing two acceptable alternatives for responding to adult requests in order to give Karl a sense of control over the situation.

e. Not allowing Karl to change his mind after he has made a choice.

f. Refraining from authoritarian responses to Karl's negative comments.

6. Specific training in social skills is highly recommended for Karl. The following are examples of structured programs:

Goldstein, A.P. (1988). *The Prepare Curriculum.* Champaign, IL: Research Press.

McGinnis, E., Goldstein, A., Sprafkin, R., Gershaw, J., & Klein, P. (1980). *Skillstreaming the Adolescent.* Champaign, IL: Research Press.

7. Involving Karl in peer tutoring situations would help promote social responsibility. The best arrangement would be to have Karl tutor a peer in areas where he has special academic strengths, such as math or science. Encouragement of leadership roles and cooperative learning situations, such as science projects, is also recommended.

8. An assignment book is necessary to help Karl organize his school work and plan long-term assignments. It would also be helpful to break long-term assignments down into small components and to monitor his progress on the components.

9. Regular home-school communication is important for maintaining a consistent behavior management program. A home-school log could be helpful to provide daily reports regarding accomplishments as well as problems. School problems should be handled within that context as much as possible rather than postponing negative consequences until Karl gets home. The following resource is recommended:

Kelley, M.L. (1990). *School-Home Notes. Promoting Children's Classroom Success.* New York: Guilford.

10. Individual psychotherapy may be helpful to develop Karl's social coping skills and to address personal issues. A concrete, behavioral approach, focusing on problem-solving skills, is likely to be most effective.

11. A parent education group is recommended for Mr. and Mrs. Ladd to develop strategies for managing

Karl's aggressive and noncompliant behavior. An example of such a program is:

Barkley, R. (1987) *Defiant Children. A Clinician's Manual for Parent Training.* New York: Guilford.

SUMMARY

Four cases illustrated procedures for scoring and interpreting the SCICA Profile and comparing SCICA results to those from the CBCL, TRF, DOF, and YSR. Patty exemplified a very active and aggressive 6-year-old girl. The SCICA Profile documented the interviewer's observations of attention problems, resistant and strange behavior, and Patty's self-reports of aggressive behavior and family problems. The SCICA results were consistent with externalizing problems reported by Patty's mother on the CBCL and her teacher on the TRF. Ratings of Patty's school behavior on the DOF corroborated reports from other informants. Patty received DSM-IV diagnoses of ADHD and ODD.

Bruce illustrated attention problems, strange behavior, thought problems, and social problems in a 9-year-old boy. The SCICA Profile documented interviewer observations of anxiousness and strange behavior, while the CBCL and TRF revealed thought problems. The DOF identified attention problems and hyperactivity that were also consistent with results on the SCICA, CBCL, and TRF. The diagnosis of a major mental disorder in Bruce's biological father and a parental divorce were important factors in his case. Although Bruce met criteria for a DSM-IV diagnosis of ADHD, such a diagnosis failed to capture his unusual thought processes and strange behavior, or the unevenness of his cognitive abilities revealed by the WISC-III.

Catherine illustrated severe internalizing problems in an 11-year-old girl, including withdrawal, anxiety, and depression. The SCICA revealed extreme withdrawal similar to that reported by Catherine's mother on the CBCL and her teacher on the TRF. Catherine's self-reports during the SCICA, as well as on the YSR, revealed anxiousness and depression, likely related to unresolved sadness about the death of her father. The TRF and DOF also revealed attention problems, although cognitive assessment showed no evidence of learning disabilities. Catherine's pattern of problems met criteria for a DSM-IV diagnosis of Dysthymia, as well as special education criteria for Serious Emotional Disturbance (SED).

Karl illustrated severe internalizing and externalizing problems in a 12-year-old boy. On the CBCL and TRF, Karl's mother and teacher reported severe aggressive and delinquent behavior. Karl's mother also reported thought problems, while his teacher reported anxiety, unhappiness, and social problems. Karl's reports of aggressive behavior and social problems during the SCICA were consistent with parent and teacher reports. The SCICA highlighted extreme conflicts with peers and school authority figures, a preoccupation with fairness, intense anger and mood swings, but a positive reaction to a behavioral point system used at home. Although Karl's self-ratings on the YSR produced high scores for externalizing problems and withdrawal, he was even more forthcoming during the SCICA. Karl met criteria for a DSM-IV diagnosis of Conduct Disorder, as well as special education criteria for SED.

Chapter 11
Answers to Commonly
Asked Questions

This chapter answers questions that may arise about the SCICA. The questions are grouped under headings pertaining to the SCICA forms, training in the use of the SCICA, administering the SCICA, relations to other assessment procedures, coordinating data from multiple sources, and relations to DSM and special education classifications. If you have a question that is not found under one heading, look under the other headings. The Table of Contents and Index may also help you find answers to questions not listed in this chapter.

SCICA PROTOCOL, SCORING FORMS, AND PROFILE

1. How does the 1994 SCICA Protocol differ from the 1990 SCIC Protocol?

Answer: Chapter 2 presents details of the SCICA Protocol and changes from the previous SCIC Protocol. The 1990 SCIC protocol was designed for ages 6-11. The 1994 SCICA protocol includes most of the same questions and tasks as the previous protocol but now designates the younger age range as 6-12. New items have been added for ages 13-18, including direct questions about somatic complaints, substance use, and trouble with the law. To make the interview easier to administer, the protocol form has been increased from four to six pages, items have been grouped into clearer configurations, and more space has been provided for interviewer notes.

2. How do the 1994 SCICA Observation and Self-Report Forms differ from the previous versions?

Answer: Chapter 2 presents the 1994 scoring forms and the specific changes from the previous SCIC versions. The main changes are: *(1)* re-wording of a few items for clarification; *(2)* the addition of three new observational and seven new self-report items for all ages; *(3)* the transfer of somatic complaints items to the end of the self-report form; *(4)* the addition of items that are scored for adolescents on the basis of direct questions; and *(5)* re-numbering of items to accommodate these changes.

3. How does the 1994 SCICA Profile differ from the previous SCIC Profile?

Answer: Chapter 4 details the construction of the 1994 SCICA Profile. It displays syndrome scales that were derived from new principal components analyses of larger samples of subjects than the previous version. The 1994 syndrome scales are designated as *Aggressive Behavior,*[SR] *Anxious,*[OB] *Anxious/Depressed,*[SR] *Attention Problems,*[OB] *Family Problems,*[SR] *Resistant,*[OB] *Strange,*[OB] and *Withdrawn.*[OB] (The superscript SR indicates syndromes derived from self-report items, while the superscript OB indicates syndromes derived from observation items.) The age range for the reference group on which T scores and percentiles are based is now 6 to 12 years instead of 6 to 11. Research is under way to provide a basis for scoring ages 13 to 18.

4. How does the 1994 SCICA computer program differ from the previous SCIC program?

Answer: The 1994 computer-scored SCICA profile is described in Chapter 4. The main differences from the pre-1994 computer program include: *(1)* new, more user friendly data entry screens and procedures; *(2)* an option for users to score interviews observed on a training tape and to compute intraclass correlations between their scores and scores assigned by experienced raters; *(3)* new, easier to use illustrated computer manual; *(4)* an option to convert data entered with the previous SCIC program to the 1994 SCICA format without re-entering the data; *(5)* an option to enter data on one occasion and to key verify them later; and *(6)* other enhancements to improve data processing and retrieval.

5. How are the open-ended items 121 and 247 figured into the scale scores?

Answer: If the interviewer enters any problems in item 121, the highest score that the interviewer gave to any of these problems (i.e., *1, 2,* or *3*) is added to the total score for the observation items. Similarly, if the interviewer enters any problems in item 247, the highest score given to any of these problems is added to the total score for the self-report items.

6. Why are there no percentiles or *T* scores for the "Other Problems" listed on the SCICA Profile?

Answer: The "Other Problems" on the SCICA Profile do not constitute a separate scale. They are merely the items that were either reported too seldom to be included in the derivation of syndromes or they did not qualify for the syndrome scales. There are thus no specific associations among them to warrant treating them as a separate scale. However, each of these problems may be important in its own right, and they are all included in the total score for either the Observation or Self-Report items.

7. Is there a short form of the SCICA that takes less time to administer?

Answer: If data from the achievement tests and/or gross motor screening tasks are not needed or will be obtained in other ways, these can be omitted, thereby shortening the SCICA by about 20 to 30 minutes. However, as a comprehensive clinical interview, the SCICA cannot be expected to take much less than about an hour.

8. Can ages 13-18 be scored on the profile designated for ages 6-12?

Answer: The syndromes, percentiles, and T scores displayed on the profile were derived from interviews with 6- to 12-year-olds. The first 227 items are scored in the same way for ages 13-18 as for ages 6-12. In addition, items 228-246 can be scored for ages 13-18 as indicated on page 5 of the Self-Report Form. However, it is not yet known whether similar syndromes and distributions of scores will be obtained for ages 13-18. Until syndromes and distributions of scores are derived from a sufficient sample of 13-18-year-olds, scores for these older ages may be displayed on the 1994 profile, as long as it is understood that no conclusions can be drawn about the degree of deviance indicated by particular syndrome or scale scores.

9. Should raw scale scores, percentiles, or T scores be used to report SCICA results?

Answer: Chapter 10 provides case illustrations for interpreting SCICA scores. Briefly, raw scores are usually preferable for statistical analyses, because they directly reflect all differences among subjects in a particular sample. Percentiles and T scores, on the other hand, are usually preferable for reporting clinical findings for individual children, because they indicate the degree of deviance on each scale in comparison with the reference sample of clinically referred children on whom the scales were derived. SCICA scores have not been obtained for large enough samples of nonreferred children to provide a basis for nonclinical norms. However, Appendix C provides mean scale scores for 53 nonreferred children that can be used to guide judgments of SCICA scale scores obtained by individual children.

10. Should extremely low scores on problem scales be considered deviant?

Answer: Extremely low scores merely reflect an absence of problems scored by the interviewer. Considering that the syndromes, percentiles, and *T* scores were derived on children referred for mental health or special education services, it is not unusual for children to obtain relatively low scores on one or more scales. Low SCICA scale scores do not necessarily mean that problems are absent in other contexts, such as the home or school.

11. How are clinical interpretations of the profile made?

Answer: The profile is designed to provide a standardized *description* of behavior, as scored by the interviewer and compared to scores from interviewers of our clinical reference sample. As such, it is to be integrated with everything else that is known about the child. Rather than being "interpreted," the information from the SCICA profile should be compared with data from other sources, such as parent and teacher reports. Specific guidelines and case illustrations are provided in Chapter 10.

ADMINISTERING THE SCICA

1. Who should administer the SCICA?

Answer: If their experience and training qualify them to administer the SCICA, people playing various roles with respect to children can appropriately administer the SCICA. Examples are clinicians who use the SCICA to evaluate children's needs for mental health or special education services; therapists who use the SCICA to provide a baseline and starting point for therapy; and forensic workers who use the SCICA with other data to provide expert opinions about custody, placement, and other decisions involving legal issues. The SCICA may also be administered by researchers who use it in conjunction with other procedures to test for etiological factors, predictors, correlates, responsiveness to treatment, and outcomes of psychopathology. And the SCICA may be administered by trainees who are learning to do clinical, special education, or forensic evaluations, treatment, or research. User qualifications for the SCICA are described on pages iii and iv and in response to question 1 under *Training*, later in this chapter.

2. At what point in the evaluation process should the SCICA be administered?

Answer: Section 6 of the SCICA Protocol provides for asking subjects about six problems that were scored 2 ("very true or often true") on the CBCL or TRF. Consequently, the SCICA is typically administered after a parent has completed the CBCL and/or a teacher has completed the TRF. To prevent the interviewer from being biased by prior knowledge of the problems reported on the CBCL and TRF, it is desirable to have an assistant enter the six selected problems in the spaces provided on the SCICA Protocol prior to the interview. The interviewer should avoid looking at them until reaching the point in the SCICA where they are to be broached to the subject. To optimize comparisons of the SCICA with the CBCL, TRF, and other assessment procedures, it is desirable to have all the instruments completed within a relatively short period, preferably within a week to a month, if possible. The SCICA and the other procedures can also be readministered during the course of interventions and as outcome measures to assess changes in behavioral/emotional problems.

3. How should the confidentiality of subjects' self-reports be protected?

Answer: The SCICA Protocol provides verbatim instructions for assuring subjects of confidentiality and for informing them that the interviewer might have to report danger or abuse to the subject or by the subject. The protocol form bearing the interviewer's notes and the subject's actual words should be kept strictly confidential in all cases. The scored rating forms and protocol should be protected in the same fashion as other confidential test data. Do *not* place the completed protocol, rating forms, or profile in school records or other locations where they might be seen by the subject's peers or other unauthorized people, or by people who lack appropriate training for using the SCICA.

4. How does administration of the SCICA differ for ages 6-12 versus 13-18?

Answer: The SCICA Protocol indicates several items that are to be omitted or added for ages 13-18. For example, the fine and gross motor screening items and achievement tests are not usually administered to 13-18-year-olds, whereas the specific questions on page 6 of the protocol are not administered to 6-12-year-olds. The Kinetic Family Drawing is standard for ages 6-12 but may be omitted for those 13-18-year-olds for whom it seems too childish or who reject it for other reasons.

5. Can the SCICA be used below age 6 or over age 18?

Answer: The SCICA may be appropriate for bright 5-year-olds and some 19-year-olds, but the farther the subject's abilities are from the 6- to 18-year age range, the less appropriate the format, items, and scoring will be.

6. Can the SCICA be used with children having physical or mental disabilities?

Answer: Unless physical or mental disabilities interfere significantly with the interviewing procedures, the SCICA should yield appropriate descriptive data on the interview behavior and self-reports of subjects with disabilities. However, it should not be surprising if certain disabilities affect problem behaviors, causing higher or lower elevations on syndrome scales than for subjects without disabilities. The SCICA is unlikely to be appropriate for subjects having mental ages below about 6 years or subjects with limited language skills that prevent them from participating appropriately in an interview.

7. What are the pros and cons of administering the optional achievement tests and motor screening tasks?

Answer: If more extensive assessments of achievement and motor functioning are not planned, these items provide economical screening assessments while also extending the sample of behavior to be rated. Because the achievement tests are school-like tasks of the sort that often challenge troubled children, they may elicit important behavior and self-reports that might otherwise not be seen during the SCICA. Unless there are compelling reasons to omit them, the achievement tests and motor screening tasks are therefore valuable parts of the SCICA for ages 6-12.

TRAINING IN USE OF THE SCICA

1. What kind of training and experience are needed to administer the SCICA?

Answer: Eligibility to use the SCICA requires supervised training in clinical interviewing of subjects in the age range for which the SCICA will be used, plus graduate training in standardized assessment commensurate with at least the Master's degree in psychology, social work, or special education, or two years of residency in psychiatry or pediatrics. This means that prospective interviewers should be experienced in conversing and interacting with subjects in sensitive, nondirective ways that encourage free expression by the subjects. Users also need to understand the SCICA's approach to standardized assessment and need considerable practice in administering and scoring the SCICA. The training videotape is designed to help interviewers reach agreement with scoring by experienced raters, as described in the following section. Trainees can also obtain valuable experience by watching videotapes of at least three of their own practice interviews, scoring them from the tapes, and having supervisors point out possibilities for improvement. This provides unparalleled opportunities for identifying the strengths and weaknesses of the trainee's interviewing skills.

2. How should the SCICA training tape be used to practice scoring?

Answer: The SCICA training tape available from the authors displays segments of interviews that were originally done with clinically referred children and that have been re-enacted by child actors to highlight observations and self-reports that should be scored. It is recommended that trainees first become fully familiar with the SCICA Manual, protocol, and scoring forms. They should then view the first interview segment and score it on the SCICA Observation and Self-Report Forms. Thereafter, they should select the training options on the SCICA computer-scoring program and enter their scores for Segment 1. By following the computer instructions, trainees can have a profile printed from their own Segment 1 scores for comparison with a profile printed from the mean Segment 1 scale scores obtained from experienced raters. For each of the interview segments, the computer-scoring program also prints out an intraclass correlation (ICC) between the trainee's scores and the mean of the scores obtained from the experienced raters. Trainees can repeatedly view and score each practice segment until their scores agree well with those of the experienced raters. Instructions that accompany the videotape provide further details of the practice procedures.

RELATIONS TO OTHER
ASSESSMENT PROCEDURES

1. How does the SCICA differ from structured and semistructured interviews designed to make DSM diagnoses?

Answer: The SCICA Protocol and rating forms were developed to tap important areas of children's functioning in ways that can be assessed in interviews. Unlike interviews whose questions and outputs are pre-determined by DSM diagnostic criteria, the SCICA's questions and output were developed by testing a variety of interview techniques, content, and scoring items to determine what data could typically be obtained from subjects in the target age range. The SCICA syndrome scales were then derived empirically from statistical analyses of the Observation and Self-Report items scored from interviews with clinically referred children. Chapter 1 details the differences between the SCICA and other interviews. When combined with data from other sources, the SCICA can be used to judge whether children meet criteria for certain DSM diagnoses.

2. Can the SCICA be used with other assessment procedures, such as ratings by informants, interviews with parents, behavioral and family assessment, medical exams, and personality, cognitive, and achievement tests?

Answer: No interview should be the sole basis for assessing behavioral/emotional problems. Instead, interviews provide samples of behavior and self-reports under a particular set of conditions. Comprehensive assessment therefore requires other types of data appropriate for the subject's age, the goal of the assessment, and the feasibility of other procedures. Ratings by informants, parent and teacher interviews, behavioral and family assessment, medical exams, and personality, cognitive, and achievement tests would all be candidate procedures. Chapter 1 describes our multiaxial assessment model for using the SCICA in conjunction with other procedures.

3. How do the items of the SCICA compare with those of the CBCL, TRF, YSR, and DOF?

Answer: Because the SCICA provides a sample of behavior and self-reports under conditions quite different from the subjects' everyday environments, it is not expected to yield data that directly parallel those of our other instruments. However, items from our other instruments that could be meaningfully scored on the basis of an interview were adapted for inclusion in the SCICA Observation and Self-Report Forms. Chapter 4 describes how SCICA items were derived from the CBCL and TRF. Other items were developed to take advantage of opportunities for interacting with and observing subjects in ways that are not feasible outside the interview. Because of the different perspectives afforded by the SCICA, CBCL, TRF, YSR, and DOF, they often yield different findings.

4. How do the SCICA scales compare with those of the CBCL, TRF, YSR, and DOF?

Answer: The syndrome scales for each instrument were derived separately from statistical analyses of large samples of subjects scored on that instrument. In addition, syndromes that had counterparts on the CBCL, TRF, and YSR were used to form cross-informant syndrome constructs that can be scored on scales from these three instruments. Chapter 4 details the derivation of syndrome scales for the SCICA. Chapter 8 compares the SCICA scales with those from the other instruments.

COORDINATING DATA
FROM MULTIPLE SOURCES

1. How are data from the SCICA coordinated with data from other sources?

Answer: According to our multiaxial model (Chapter 1), comprehensive clinical assessments include data from parents, teachers, tests, biomedical procedures, and direct assessment of the subject. Direct assessment may include the SCICA, plus the DOF and YSR. If a subject is assessed with our other instruments, the scores on the parallel scales can be compared to identify problem areas that consistently show deviance across all sources of data versus those that show major discrepancies. If multiple sources of data show similar kinds of deviance, this indicates that the subject's problems are likely to be consistent across contexts. A uniform cross-situational approach is therefore likely to be appropriate for modifying the subject's overall adaptive pattern. The case illustrations in Chapter 10 provide detailed examples of how multiple sources of assessment data can be coordinated to identify consistencies and inconsistencies in the subject's functioning.

2. What if there are differences between the patterns of problems obtained from the SCICA versus those obtained from the CBCL, TRF, YSR, or DOF?

Answer: Discrepancies between findings from different assessment procedures can guide users in seeking further information. For example, if the SCICA scale scores differ markedly from the corresponding CBCL scale scores, the analogous TRF and/or DOF scales can be examined to determine whether their results are more similar to the CBCL or SCICA findings. If the TRF and/or DOF findings are consistent with the SCICA but not with the CBCL, parents should be interviewed to determine whether the behavior they see differs from what was observed in the interview and school, or whether they have unusual standards for judging or reporting behavior. It is especially desirable to obtain CBCLs from both parents or other combinations of household members to determine whether only one family informant is discrepant from other sources or whether both are. If a subject has multiple teachers, it is similarly desirable to have separate TRFs to identify consistencies and inconsistencies among teacher's reports.

RELATIONS TO DSM AND
SPECIAL EDUCATION CLASSIFICATIONS

1. How can the SCICA contribute to DSM diagnoses?

Answer: Because the DSM criteria are not defined by specific assessment operations, any type and source of data may be relevant to judging whether each criterial feature of a DSM diagnostic category is present. The SCICA provides scores for many specific problems that have counterparts in the DSM criteria. When used with data from other sources, scores on the SCICA items provide a basis for judging whether the corresponding DSM criteria are met.

2. How can the SCICA be used in determining eligibility for special education according to administrative classifications of disabilities, such as those based on the Individuals with Disabilities Education Act?

Answer: Like the DSM, administrative classifications for special education are not defined in terms of specific procedures for assessing children. However, the SCICA and related procedures provide an empirical basis for judging whether children have the kinds of problems for which particular kinds of special educational services are intended. The SCICA can also be combined with other assessment procedures to determine whether students meet eligibility criteria for special education under the category of Serious Emotional Disturbance (SED) (McConaughy & Ritter, in press). Chapter 10 provides case illustrations of students who meet SED criteria for special education.

REFERENCES

Abramowitz, M., & Stegun, I.A. (1968). *Handbook of mathematical functions.* Washington, D.C.: National Bureau of Standards.

Achenbach, T.M. (1966). The classification of children's psychiatric symptoms: A factor-analytic study. *Psychological Monographs, 80* (No. 615).

Achenbach, T.M. (1991a). *Integrative guide for the 1991 CBCL/4-18, YSR, and TRF profiles.* Burlington, VT: University of Vermont Department of Psychiatry.

Achenbach, T.M. (1991b). *Manual for the Child Behavior Checklist/4-18 and 1991 Profile.* Burlington, VT: University of Vermont Department of Psychiatry.

Achenbach, T.M. (1991c). *Manual for the Teacher's Report Form and 1991 Profile.* Burlington, VT: University of Vermont Department of Psychiatry.

Achenbach, T.M. (1991d). *Manual for the Youth Self-Report and 1991 Profile.* Burlington, VT: University of Vermont Department of Psychiatry.

Achenbach, T.M. (1993). *Empirically based taxonomy: How to use syndromes and profile types derived from the CBCL/4-18, TRF, and YSR.* Burlington, VT: University of Vermont Department of Psychiatry.

Achenbach, T.M., & Edelbrock, C. (1981). Behavioral problems and competencies reported by parents of normal and disturbed children aged four to sixteen. *Monographs of the Society for Research in Child Development, 46*(Serial No. 188).

Achenbach, T.M., McConaughy, S.H., & Howell, C.T. (1987). Child/ adolescent behavioral and emotional problems: Implications of cross-informant correlations for situational specificity. *Psychological Bulletin, 101,* 213-232.

AERA, APA, & NCME. (1985). *Standards for educational and psychological testing.* Washington, DC: American Psychological Association.

Ambrosini, P.J., Metz, C., Prabucki, K., & Lee, J. (1989). Videotape reliability of the third revised edition of the K-SADS. *Journal of the American Academy of Child and Adolescent Psychiatry, 28,* 723-728.

American Psychiatric Association. (1980, 1987, 1994). *Diagnostic and statistical manual of mental disorders (3rd ed., 3rd rev. ed., 4th ed.).* Washington, D.C.: Author.

Angold, A., & Costello, E.J. (1993). *A test-retest reliability study of child-reported psychiatric symptoms and diagnoses using the Child and Adolescent Psychiatric Assessment (CAPA).* Durham, NC: Duke University, Department of Psychiatry.

Angold, A., Cox, A., Prendergast, M., Rutter, M., & Simonoff, E. (1987). *Child and Adolescent Psychiatric Assessment (CAPA)*. Durham, NC: Duke University, Department of Psychiatry.

Biederman, J., Faraone, S.V., Doyle, A., Lehman, B.K., Kraus, I., Perrin, J., & Tsuang, M.T. (1993). Convergence of the Child Behavior Checklist with structured interview-based psychiatric diagnoses of ADHD children with and without comorbidity. *Journal of Child Psychology and Psychiatry, 34*, 1241-1251.

Bird, H.R., Canino, G., Rubio-Stipec, M., Gould, M.S., Ribera, J., Sesman, M., Woodbury, M., Huertas-Goldman, S., Pagan, A., Sanchez-Lacay, A., & Moscoso, M. (1988). Estimates of the prevalence of childhood maladjustment in a community survey in Puerto Rico. *Archives of General Psychiatry, 45*, 1120-1126.

Bird, H.R., Gould, M.S., & Staghezza, B. (1992). Aggregating data from multiple informants in child psychiatry epidemiological research. *Journal of the American Academy of Child and Adolescent Psychiatry, 31*, 78-85.

Boyle, M.H., Offord, D.R., Racine, Y., Sanford, M., Szatmari, P., Fleming, J.E., & Price-Munn, N. (1993). Evaluation of the Diagnostic Interview for Children and Adolescents for use in general population samples. *Journal of Abnormal Child Psychology, 21*, 663-681.

Burns, B.J., Angold, A., Macgruder-Habib, K., Costello, E.J., & Patrick, M.K.S. (1992). *The Child and Adolescent Services Assessment (CASA)*. Durham, NC: Duke University Department of Psychiatry.

Burns, R.C. (1982). *Self-growth in families: Kinetic family drawings (K-F-D) research and application*. New York: Brunner/Mazel.

Cohen, J. (1988). *Statistical power analysis for the behavioral sciences* (2nd ed.). New York: Academic Press.

Costello, A.J., Edelbrock, C., Dulcan, M.K., Kalas, R., & Klaric, S.H. (1984). *Report on the Diagnostic Interview Schedule for Children (DISC)*. Pittsburgh, PA: University of Pittsburgh, Department of Psychiatry.

Costello, E.J. (1989). Developments in child psychiatric epidemiology. *Journal of the American Academy of Child and Adolescent Psychiatry, 28*, 836-841.

Costello, E.J., Burns, B.J., Angold, A., & Leaf, P.J. (1993). How can epidemiology improve mental health services for children and adolescents? *Journal of the American Academy of Child and Adolescent Psychiatry, 32*, 1106-1113.

Crocker, L., & Algina, J. (1986). *Introduction to classical and modern test theory*. New York: Holt, Rinehart, & Winston.

Cronbach, L.J. (1951). Coefficient alpha and the internal structure of tests. *Psychometrika, 16*, 297-334.

Dunn, L.C., & Markwardt, F.C. (1970, 1989). *Peabody Individual Achievement Test*. Circle Pines, MN: American Guidance Service.

Edelbrock, C., & Costello, A.J. (1988). Convergence between statistically derived behavior problem syndromes and child psychiatric diagnoses. *Journal of Abnormal Child Psychology, 16*, 219-231.

Edelbrock, C., Costello, A.J., Dulcan, M.K., Conover, N.C., & Kalas, R. (1986). Parent-child agreement on child psychiatric symptoms assessed via structured interview. *Journal of Child Psychology and Psychiatry, 27*, 181-190.

Edelbrock, C., Costello, A.J., Dulcan, M.K., Kalas, R., & Conover, N.C. (1985). Age differences in the reliability of the psychiatric interview of the child. *Child Development, 56*, 265-275.

Einhorn, H.J. (1988). Diagnosis and causality in clinical and statistical prediction. In D.C. Turk (Ed.), *Reasoning, inference, and judgment in clinical psychology*. New York: Free Press.

Garbarino, J., & Scott, F.M. (1989). *What children can tell us*. San Francisco: Jossey-Bass.

Gorsuch, R.L. (1983). *Factor analysis* (2nd ed.). Hillsdale, NJ: Erlbaum.

Gould, M.S., Bird, H., & Jaramillo, B.S. (1993). Correspondence between statistically derived behavior problem syndromes and child psychiatric diagnoses in a community sample. *Journal of Abnormal Child Psychology, 21*, 287-313.

Gutterman, E.M., O'Brien, J.D., & Young, J.G. (1987). Structured diagnostic interviews for children and adolescents: Current status and future directions. *Journal of the American Academy of Child and Adolescent Psychiatry, 26*, 621-630.

Herjanic, B., & Reich, W. (1982). Development of a structured psychiatric interview for children: Agreement between child and parent on individual symptoms. *Journal of Abnormal Child Psychology, 10*, 307-24.

Hodges, K. (1993). Structured interviews for assessing children. *Journal of Child Psychology and Psychiatry, 34*, 49-68.

Hodges, K., Cools, J., & McKnew, D. (1989). Test-retest reliability of a clinical research interview for children: The Child Assessment Schedule. *Psychological Assessment, 1*, 317-322.

Hodges, K., Gordon, Y., & Lennon, M. (1990). Parent-child agreement on symptoms assessed via a clinical research interview for children: The Child Assessment Schedule (CAS). *Journal of Child Psychology and Psychiatry, 31*, 427-436.

Hodges, K., McKnew, D., Cytryn, L., Stern, L., & Kline, J. (1982). The Child Assessment Schedule (CAS) Diagnostic Interview: A report on reliability and validity. *Journal of the American Academy of Child Psychiatry, 21*, 468-73.

Hollingshead, A.B. (1975). *Four factor index of social status.* New Haven, CT: Unpublished paper. Yale University, Department of Sociology.

Hughes, J., & Baker, D.B. (1990). *The clinical child interview.* New York: Guilford Press.

Hughes, J.N. (1989). The child interview. *School Psychology Review, 18,* 247-259.

Individuals with Disabilities Education Act. (1990). *Public Law* 101-476. 20 U.S.C. § 1401.

Jensen, P., Roper, M., Fisher, P., & Piacentini, J. (1994). *Test-retest reliability of the Diagnostic Interview Schedule for Children (ver. 2.1): Parent, child, and combined algorithms.* Manuscript submitted for publication.

John, K., Gammon, G.D., Prusoff, B.A., & Warner, V. (1987). The Social Adjustment Inventory for Children and Adolescents (SAICA): Testing of a new semistructured interview. *Journal of the American Academy of Child and Adolescent Psychiatry, 26,* 898-911.

Kaufman, A.S., & Kaufman, N.L (1983). *Kaufman Assessment Battery for Children.* Circle Pines, MN: American Guidance Service.

Kaufman, A.S., & Kaufman, N.L. (1985). *Kaufman Test of Educational Achievement.* Circle Pines, MN: American Guidance Service.

Kestenbaum, C.J., & Bird, H.R. (1978). A reliability study of the Mental Health Assessment Form for school-age children. *Journal of the American Academy of Child Psychiatry, 17,* 338-347.

Koppitz, E.M. (1975). *The Bender Gestalt Test for young children* (Vol. II). New York: Grune & Stratton.

Kovacs, M. (1983). *The Interview Schedule for Children (ISC).* Pittsburgh: University of Pittsburgh, Department of Psychiatry.

Loeber, R.,, Green, S.M., Lahey, B.B., & Stouthamer-Loeber, M. (1989). Optimal informants on child disruptive behaviors. *Development and Psychopathology, 1,* 317-337.

Mattison, R.E., & Bagnato, S.J. (1987). Empirical measurement of over-anxious disorder in boys 8 to 12 years old. *Journal of the American Academy of Child and Adolescent Psychiatry, 26,* 536-540.

McConaughy, S.H. (1993a). Advances in empirically based assessment of children's behavioral and emotional problems. *School Psychology Review, 22,* 285-307.

McConaughy, S.H. (1993b). Evaluating behavioral and emotional disorders with the CBCL, TRF, and YSR cross-informant scales. *Journal of Emotional and Behavioral Disorders, 1,* 40-52.

McConaughy, S.H., & Achenbach, T.M. (1990). *Guide for the Semistructured Clinical Interview for Children Aged 6-11.* Burlington, VT: University of Vermont Department of Psychiatry.

McConaughy, S.H., Mattison, R.E., & Peterson, R.L. (1994). Behavioral/emotional problems of children with serious emotional disturbance and learning disabilities. *School Psychology Review, 23,* 81-98.

McConaughy, S.H., & Ritter, D. (in press). Multidimensional assessment of emotional or behavioral disorders. In A. Thomas & J. Grimes (Eds.), *Best practices in school psychology III.* Washington, D.C.: National Association of School Psychologists.

McConaughy, S.H., & Skiba, R.J. (1993). Comorbidity of externalizing and internalizing problems. *School Psychology Review, 22,* 421-436.

Piacentini, J.C., Cohen, P., & Cohen, J. (1992). Combining discrepant diagnostic information from multiple sources. Are complex algorithms better than simple ones? *Journal of Abnormal Child Psychology, 20,* 51-63.

Puig-Antich, J., & Chambers, W. (1978). *The Schedule for Affective Disorders and Schizophrenia for School-aged Children (Kiddie-SADS).* New York: New York State Psychiatric Institute.

Reich, W., & Welner, Z. (1992). *DICA-R-C. DSM-III-R version. Revised version of DICA for children ages 6-12.* St. Louis, MO: Washington University, Department of Psychiatry.

Rey, J.M., & Morris-Yates, A. (1992). Diagnostic accuracy in adolescents of several depression rating scales extracted from a general purpose behavior checklist. *Journal of Affective Disorders, 26,* 7-16.

Rey, J.M., Morris-Yates, A., & Stanislaw, H. (1992). Measuring the accuracy of diagnostic tests using Receiver Operating Characteristics (ROC) analysis. *International Journal of Methods in Psychiatric Research, 2,* 39-50.

Robins, L.N., Helzer, J.E., Cottler, L., & Goldring, E. (1989). *NIMH Diagnostic Interview Schedule, Version III Revised (DSM-III-R).* St. Louis, MO: Washington University Department of Psychiatry.

Rutter, M., & Graham, P. (1968). The reliability and validity of the psychiatric assessment of the child: I. Interview with the child. *British Journal of Psychiatry, 114,* 563-579.

Sakoda, J.M., Cohen, B.H., & Beall, G. (1954). Test of significance for a series of statistical tests. *Psychological Bulletin, 51,* 172-175.

SAS Institute. (1990). *SAS/STAT User's Guide, Release 6.04 Edition.* Cary, NC: SAS Institute.

Shaffer, D. (1992). *Diagnostic Interview Schedule for Children, Version 2.3.* New York: Columbia University Division of Child Psychiatry.

Shaffer, D., Schwab-Stone, M., Fisher, P., Davies, M., Piacentini, J., & Gioia, P. (1988). *A revised version of the Diagnostic Interview Schedule for Children*. New York: Columbia University Division of Child Psychiatry.

Snook, S.C., & Gorsuch, R.L. (1989). Component analysis versus common factor analysis: A Monte Carlo study. *Psychological Bulletin, 106*, 148-154.

Verhulst, F.C., Akkerhuis, G.W., & Althaus, M. (1985). Mental health in Dutch children: (I) A cross-cultural comparison. *Acta Psychiatrica Scandinavica, 72*(Suppl. 323).

Verhulst, F.C., Versluis-den Bieman, M.S., van der Ende, J., Berden, G.F.M.G., & Sanders-Woudstra, J. (1990). Problem behavior in international adoptees: III. Diagnosis of child psychiatric disorder. *Journal of the American Academy of Child and Adolescent Psychiatry, 29*, 420-428.

Wechsler, D.C. (1991). *Wechsler Intelligence Scale for Children-Third edition*. San Antonio, TX: Psychological Corporation.

Wechsler, D.C. (1992). *Wechsler Individual Achievement Test*. San Antonio, TX: Psychological Corporation.

Weinstein, S.R., Noam, G.G., Grimes, K., Stone, K., & Schwab-Stone, M. (1990). Convergence of DSM-III diagnoses and self-reported symptoms in child and adolescent inpatients. *Journal of the American Academy of Child and Adolescent Psychiatry, 29*, 627-634.

Wilkinson, G.S. (1993). *Wide Range Achievement Test*. Wilmington, DL: Wide Range, Inc..

Witt, J.C., Cavell, T.A., Carey, M.P., & Martens, B. (1988). Child self- report: Interviewing techniques and rating scales. In E.S. Shapiro & R.R. Kratochwill (Eds.), *Behavioral assessment in schools: Conceptual foundations and practical applications*. New York: Guilford Press.

Woodcock, R.E., & Johnson, M.B. (1989). *Woodcock-Johnson Psychoeducational Battery-Revised*. Hingham, MA: Teaching Resources Corp.

World Health Organization, (1992). *Mental disorders: Glossary and guide to their classification in accordance with the Tenth Revision of the International Classification of Diseases* (10th ed.). Geneva: Author.

Young, J.G., O'Brien, J.D., Gutterman, E.M., & Cohen, P. (1987). Research on the clinical interview. *Journal of the American Academy of Child and Adolescent Psychiatry, 26*, 613-620.

APPENDIX A
INSTRUCTIONS FOR SCORING THE SCICA
OBSERVATION AND SELF-REPORT FORMS

Following administration of the SCICA, the interviewer (or a videotape rater) scores the subject on the *SCICA Observation* and *Self-Report Forms*.

Scoring the SCICA Observation Form

Items on pages 1 and 2 of the SCICA Observation Form describe aspects of the subject's behavior, affect, and interaction style observed during the interview. Each observation item is scored on a 4-point scale according to the following instructions:

For each item that describes the subject's behavior during the interview, circle:
0 *if there was no occurrence;*
1 *if there was a very slight or ambiguous occurrence;*
2 *if there was a definite occurrence with mild to moderate intensity and less than 3 minutes duration; and*
3 *if there was a definite occurrence with severe intensity or 3 or more minutes duration.*

The interviewer's or rater's notes on the SCICA Protocol provide a basis for remembering the observations to be scored. Items should be scored to reflect actual observations made during the interview. A rater should score only the item that most specifically describes a particular observation. For example, several observation items describe attention problems or hyperactivity, such as *31. Doesn't concentrate or pay attention for long on tasks, questions, or topics; 32. Doesn't sit still, restless, or hyperactive; 33. Easily distracted by external stimuli; 38. Fidgets; 40. Frequently off task; 53. Lapses in attention; 64. Needs repetition of instructions or questions;* and *89. Stares blankly.* If a subject exhibits any such problems during the SCICA, a rater should score the one item that best fits the actual behavior observed. A rater may score more than one item only if the subject exhibits more than one different kind of problem, such as difficulty concentrating at certain times, being off-task at other times, and being restless throughout the interview. A rater should avoid scoring more than one item for the same observation.

Observation items should not be scored solely on the basis of inferences made from the subject's self-reports, drawings, or play. For example, a subject may describe feelings of sadness associated with past events, but not appear unhappy or sad during the interview (e.g., by looking glum or crying). In this case, a rater should score item *147. Reports being unhappy, sad, or depressed* on the Self-Report Form, but not item *107. Unhappy, sad, or depressed* on the Observation Form. On the other hand, a subject may be restless or have trouble sitting still during the interview, but deny having such problems when directly questioned about reports by parents or teachers in Section 6 of the SCICA Protocol. In this case, a rater should score the subject on item *32. Doesn't sit still, restless, or hyperactive* on the Observation Form, but not item *145. Reports being unable to sit still, being restless, or hyperactive* on the Self-Report Form.

The intensity of the occurrence and the 3-minute duration are guidelines for choosing between ratings of *1, 2,* and *3.* If it is unclear whether a particular behavior occurred, or if there was only a slight occurrence, then the relevant item should be scored *1.* If a particular behavior definitely occurred with mild to moderate intensity and less than 3 minutes over the course of the interview, the relevant item should be scored *2.* To be scored *3,* a particular behavior should have occurred with severe intensity, or occurred for 3 or more minutes over a given interval, or occurred intermittently for a total of 3 or more minutes throughout the interview.

Guidelines for Scoring Specific Items of the Observation Form. Guidelines for scoring specific items on the Observation Form are summarized below. Users can refer to these guidelines when questions arise during scoring. Several guidelines are intended to help users differentiate between similar items. It is not necessary to memorize the guidelines for scoring the SCICA.

5. Apathetic or unmotivated. Score for an "I don't care attitude" or an apathetic approach to questions or tasks, or when the subject does not bother to try to answer questions or perform tasks. Score *1* if the behavior does not begin until late in the interview. Score item 80 for a subject who seems overtired or fatigued and item 106 for underactive or slow moving.

7. Asks for feedback on performance (describe). Includes requests for feedback during achievement testing. A score of *3* should be reserved for very persistent or intense requests for feedback or frequent requests that total ≥3 minutes duration.

8. Attempts to leave for reasons other than toilet and *55. Leaves room during session to go to toilet*. Score *2* for a single occurrence with duration <5 minutes; score *3* for more than one occurrence or duration of ≥5 minutes. (This item diverges from the 3-minute duration criterion.)

9. Avoids eye contact. Score *1* if avoiding eye contact occurs *only* during the "warm up" period of approximately the first 10 minutes of the session.

10. Irresponsible, destructive, or dangerous behavior (describe). Score for destroying things during the interview (e.g., ripping paper or drawings, breaking pencils), doing physically dangerous behaviors (e.g., climbing up on high furniture, poking pencils at wall plugs), or getting into the interviewer's belongings (e.g., taking objects off interviewer's desk, opening desk drawers or file cabinets).

11. Behaves like opposite sex. Score for a boy who acts effeminate in voice or gestures or a girl who wants to be called by a boy's name or acts tough and masculine. Do not score for the boy who has feminine physical features or the girl who looks "tomboyish".

17. Can't get mind of certain thoughts; obsessions (describe). For a score of *3*, the content of expressed thoughts should be quite specific and unusual regarding an activity or object. There must be explicit preoccupation with a specific idea that intrudes into other topics. Scores of *1* and *2* can be used when there is doubt about the specificity of the preoccupation, or when the intensity or duration is not extreme.

20. Complains of dizziness, headaches, or other somatic problems during session (describe). Score for complaints of aches or pains that occur during the session and have no known medical or physical cause. Do not score for bumping an elbow. Do score for complaints of migraines or hand hurting while drawing or writing. The interviewer can use historical or medical data from clinical records or parent interviews to decide whether or not to score this item. For example, if the interviewer learned that the subject had a headache because of a need for glasses, or the subject wasn't feeling well due to a cold or flu, this item should be scored *0*.

21. Complains of tasks being too hard or becomes upset by tasks. Score for complaints that questions or tasks, such as drawings or tests, are too hard. Score also for obvious signs of frustration with a task or questions.

22. Concrete thinking. Score if the subject has difficulty generalizing from specific instances or is unusually literal in responding to questions.

23. *Confused or seems to be in a fog*. Score for behaviors that suggest confused thinking or confusion about the interview process. Score item 46 for difficulty remembering facts or details. Score item 86 for slowness in responding to questions or assigned tasks. Also see items 30, 31, or 45 for more specific observations.

30. *Disjointed or tangential conversation*. Score when the subject makes comments that are off the specific topic of conversation, or when the subject's conversation strays from the main topic.

31. *Doesn't concentrate or pay attention for long on tasks, questions, topics*. Score for problems with concentration or a short attention span, but not for intermittent lapses in attention (item 53) or distractibility (item 33). Also score when a subject has difficulty returning to a task or when there is no recovery of attention back to the original task once attention has wandered. Score item 40 for off-task behavior.

32. *Doesn't sit still, restless, or hyperactive*. Score *1* if restlessness does not begin until late in session. Score for behaviors such as squirming in seat, frequently changing position, swinging feet, or draping body across seat. Score item 38 for fidgeting, item 67 for out of seat behavior, and item 49 for more general impulsive behavior. If the subject is restless in seat and gets out of seat to walk around the room while talking, then both items 32 and 67 may be scored.

33. *Easily distracted by external stimuli*. Score when a subject is distracted by a specific object, noise, or visual stimulus that takes the subject off task. Examples are hearing noises or voices outside of the interview room, seeing planes flying by the window, hearing or seeing cars in the parking lot, and asking about pictures or objects in the room.

38. *Fidgets*. Score for non-purposeful activity with hands that includes an object. Examples are twirling hair, tapping pencils, picking at paper edges, and twisting the sleeve of a shirt.

39. *Fine motor difficulty (describe)*. Score for uncoordinated hand movements when drawing or writing, problems manipulating pencils, heavy pressure on pencil, awkward pencil grasp, etc. Score item 60 for messy work. Score items 39 and 60 when the subject clearly has fine motor difficulties and produces messy work. Score item 60 only when the subject's work is messy, but the subject does not display fine motor problems as described above.

40. Frequently off-task. Score when a subject does something that is different from what the interviewer requests or a given task requires. Do not score for a subject who is inattentive, but stays on task. Score item 31 for problems concentrating or inattentiveness.

43. Guesses a lot; does not think out answers or strategies. Score when a subject guesses on achievement tests or in responding to questions regarding factual information.

44. Difficulty expressing self verbally (describe). Do not score for poor grammar, limited vocabulary, or using gestures to accompany speech. Score for problems in verbal fluency or communicating meaning or using actions or gestures in place of verbal descriptions.

45. Difficulty understanding language (describe). Score for difficulty understanding the meaning of questions or the interviewer's conversation or need to have questions simplified. Score item 29 for difficulty following directions on drawing tasks or achievement tests. Do not score for problems that appear to be related to hearing loss. Hearing problems should be listed under item 121.

48. Impatient. Score when the subject's comments or behaviors imply a time pressure, such as when a subject wants to know when the interview will be finished or when he/she will be picked up. Score item 112 if the subject expresses a desire to quit the interview or a specific task, such as items on achievement tests.

49. Impulsive or acts without thinking. Score for immediate actions or responses that seem impulsive, such as grabbing things or shifting from one action to another. Score item 115 for a subject who has a hurried approach to a specific task, such as the writing sample, drawing, or achievement subtests.

52. Lacks self-confidence or makes self-deprecating remarks. Score for comments or behaviors that demonstrate lack of confidence or uncertainty about ability. Examples are saying, "I can't do this," or "I'm no good at drawing," or "I am so stupid". Score item 50 for more specific behaviors that indicate fear of making mistakes, such as fearing mistakes on achievement tests.

53. Lapses in attention. Score for situations when a subject's attention intermittently lapses, resulting in an interruption in behavior or conversation. Score item 31 for problems concentrating or inattention.

54. Laughs inappropriately. Score when a subject's affect is different from what would normally be expected or is inappropriate for the content of the conversation, such as laughing when describing violence.

60. Messy work. Score for written work or drawings that are illegible, messy, or sloppy considering the subject's age. Score item 115 for a hurried or careless approach to writing or drawings. Score item 39 for fine motor problems. Item 60 may be scored along with items 39 and/or 115 if fine motor problems and/or working carelessly result in a messy work product.

61. Misbehaves, taunts, or tests the limits. Score when a subject breaks the rules or limits set by the interviewer, such as grabbing toys or papers when told not to. Score item 105 for attempts to manipulate the interviewer or interview tasks.

64. Needs repetition of instructions or questions. Score when a subject needs questions or directions repeated. Do not score for repetitions made because the subject was resistant or uncooperative. Score item 63 for subjects who need coaxing or item 76 for resistant or uncooperative behavior.

65. Nervous, highstrung, or tense and **66. Nervous movements.** Score for nervous, jumpy, overdriven, or "uptight" behavior or demeanor or a general feeling of nervous tension from the subject. Score item 66 for more specific behaviors, such as twitching, eye blinks, or facial tics. Score item 104 for tremors or shaking hands or fingers. Score item 101 for tension that reflects angry mood. Score item 32 for problems sitting still or restless behavior.

69. Perseverates. Score if the subject persists with a specific topic or theme after it has been adequately covered or when the interviewer has tried to change the topic. The repetitious theme may reappear after conversation has moved to a new topic. Score item 17 for obsessive thoughts about unusual topics or topics that intrude into other topics.

72. Refuses to talk and **73. Reluctant to discuss feelings or personal issues.** Score item 72 for a subject who clearly refuses to talk. Score item 73 for a subject who does talk, but is reluctant to discuss certain issues or topics.

75. Repeats certain acts over and over; compulsions (describe). Score for repetitive, purposeless behaviors, such as touching things over and over, rubbing hands or arms on the table, or repetitively straightening things on the interviewer's desk.

76. *Resistant or refuses to comply (describe)*. Score for resistance or failure to comply with task demands within the interview, such as resisting or refusing to do achievement tests or the Kinetic Family Drawing. Score item 61 when a subject tests rules or expectations regarding behavior.

79. *Secretive*. Do not score merely for reluctance to discuss feelings or personal issues, which are covered by item 73.

80. *Seems overtired or fatigued*. Score when a subject looks physically tired or sleepy. Score a *1* if the behavior does not begin until late in the interview. Score item 5 for being apathetic or unmotivated and item 106 for underactive or slow moving.

83. *Self-conscious or easily embarrassed*. Score for behaviors indicating being self-conscious or embarrassed, such as blushing, looking apologetic, sheepishness, or unusual sensitivity.

85. *Shy*. Score for shy demeanor. Do not score for characteristics that are covered more specifically by other items, such as item 52 for lacks confidence, item 86 for slow to respond, or item 87 for slow to warm up.

87. *Slow to warm up*. Score for a subject who eventually does warm up or who seems withdrawn only in the beginning of the interview (roughly the first 5 to 10 minutes). Score item 114 for a subject who appears withdrawn or who fails to warm up.

89. *Stares blankly*. Score when a subject's eyes are not focusing on anything. Score item 53 when the subject's attention lapses in a way that disrupts his or her behavior, but he/she is looking at something. Score item 9 for avoiding eye contact.

91. *Strange behavior* and **92. *Strange ideas*.** Score item 91 for behavior that seems very unusual. Score item 92 for very unusual ideas, delusional fantasies or ideas, paranoid ideation, or strange beliefs. Scores for item 92 must be based on what the subject says, rather than on inferences from the subject's drawings or play. If the behavior or ideas are more specifically covered by another item, score the more specific item instead.

93. *Stubborn, sullen, or irritable*. Score for a generally stubborn, sullen, or irritable demeanor. Score item 96 for sulking as a specific reaction during the interview.

96. *Sulks*. Score for sulking when it is a reaction to something that occurs during the interview. Score item 93 for more general demeanor of stubbornness, sullenness, or irritability.

99. Talks aloud to self. Score for speech directed toward the self, and not toward the interviewer. Score when a subject is thinking aloud and it is clear that the purpose of the subject's comments are not meant to communicate with the interviewer. Score *1* for whispering to self during writing, drawing, or play. Do not score for talking aloud during the Kinetic Family Drawing if a subject's comments are intended to describe the drawing to the interviewer as the subject is drawing.

102. Too concerned with neatness, cleanliness, or order. Score for behaviors such as excessive tidying of interview materials, expressed concerns about getting hands or clothing dirty, etc. Do not score only for erasures while drawing or writing, unless erasures are clearly due to overconcern for neatness. Score item 34 for erasures or crossing out during writing or drawing.

103. Too fearful or anxious. Score for a subject who expresses fears of the interviewer or interview situation or who appears fearful.

105. Tries to control or manipulate interviewer. Score when a subject tries to control the course of the interview questions or tasks or tries to change the task demands, or tries to get the interviewer to do something different. Examples are when a subject wants to ask the questions instead of the interviewer or wants to administer achievement tests to the interviewer. Score item 61 for misbehavior or testing the limits or rules.

106. Underactive or slow moving. Score when a subject's physical movements are slowed down, such as in writing, drawing, or walking across the room. Score *1* if the behavior does not begin until late in the session. Score item 5 for subjects who seem apathetic or unmotivated or item 80 for subjects who seem overtired or fatigued.

112. Wants to quit or does quit tasks. Score when a subject expresses a desire to quit a task (e.g., saying "Can we stop now?"), or score when a subject actually does quit a task or the interview.

114. Withdrawn, doesn't get involved with interviewer. Score when a subject remains uninvolved, distant, does not interact throughout the interview, or withdraws off and on throughout the interview. Score item 87 a subject who is slow to warm up.

115. Works quickly and carelessly. Score when a subject approaches a specific task quickly or carelessly. Score item 49 when hurriedness or impulsivity are more general behaviors during the interview.

116. Worries. Score only for worries that the subject expresses about the interview or that occur during the session. Examples are a subject worrying about when or if his/her parent will be coming back, worrying about what interview questions or tasks require, or worrying whether the interview will result in missing some other desired activity.

117. Yawns. Score *1* for one or two definite or ambiguous yawns; score *2* or *3* for persistent yawning.

Scoring the SCICA Self-Report Form

Self-report items 122-235 on pages 3 and 4 of the SCICA Self-Report Form are scored on the same 4-point scale used for scoring observations as follows:

For each item that describes the subject's conversation during the session, circle:
0 if there was no occurrence;
1 if there was a very slight or ambiguous occurrence;
2 if there was a definite occurrence with mild to moderate intensity and less than 3 minutes duration; and
3 if there was a definite occurrence with severe intensity or 3 or more minutes duration.

A rater should score only the item that most specifically describes the subject's conversation during the interview. Ratings of *1*, *2*, and *3* are used to score the intensity and duration of the subject's self-reports during the session. If a particular problem is discussed only briefly or in an ambiguous manner, then the relevant item is scored *1*. Judgments of intensity for scores of *2* or *3* should be made according to how a particular problem is reported by the subject, not according to the interviewer's judgment of the severity of the problem. The 3-minute duration refers to the length of time a particular problem is discussed during the interview. For example, a subject may report a problem, such as physically attacking another child with a weapon, but discuss the problem in a nonchalant manner and for less than 3 minutes. In this case, a rater should assign a score of *2* to item *188. Reports physically attacking people, including siblings*, even though the rater may judge what the subject reports to reflect a severe problem. To be scored *3*, a problem must be reported as a severe concern to the subject, or must be discussed for 3 or more minutes over a given interval, or discussed intermittently throughout the interview for a total of 3 or more minutes.

In Section 6 of the SCICA Protocol, the interviewer asks the subject about specific problems reported by parents and/or teachers. If a subject acknowledges such a problem in Section 6 without further elaboration, the item is scored *1*. If a subject elaborates on the problem, or has discussed the problem in previous sections, the relevant item should be scored *2* or *3* depending on the intensity or duration of the self-report. Finally, if a subject reports a problem that clearly ended more than 6 months prior to the interview, or if the subject never discusses a problem in the interview, the corresponding item is scored *0*. When a subject reports problems that clearly occurred more than 6 months prior to the interview, such as sexual abuse, the interviewer may still score other items that reflect current self-reported emotional reactions to the problems, such as *147. Reports being unhappy, sad, or depressed* or *214. Reports worrying*.

Items 122-227 are scored for all ages. For ages 6-12, items 228-235 on page 4 of the SCICA Self-Report Form describe somatic complaints that are scored according to the same criteria as used for other items. For ages 13-18, items 228-246 on page 5 describe somatic complaints, substance use, and trouble with the law. These items are scored as follows: If a subject answers "no" to a question, score the item *0*; if a subject answers "yes" to a question, score the item according to the specific anchor points designated for choosing between ratings of *1*, *2*, and *3*; if a subject refuses to answer a question, score the item *4*. The numbering of items 228-246 for ages 13-18 corresponds to questions listed in Section 9 on page 6 of the SCICA Protocol. Additional self-reported problems not covered by items 122-246 should be recorded in the spaces under item 247 and scored according to the criteria for items 122-227.

Guidelines for Scoring Specific Items of the Self-Report Form. Guidelines for scoring specific items on the Self-Report Form are summarized below. Users can refer to these guidelines when questions arise during scoring. Several guidelines are intended to help users differentiate between similar items. It is not necessary to memorize the guidelines for scoring the SCICA.

126. Reports being beaten up by others including siblings (exclude parents). Do not score reports of getting hit if the subject is not beaten up. Score item 174 for getting hit or teased.

130. Reports being disobedient at home and *131. Reports being disobedient at school.* Score for reports of disobedience, breaking home or school rules, or for reports of consequences of behavior that are clearly due to violations of home or school rules, such as getting sent to room, getting time-outs, getting detentions, or being sent to principal's office.

135. Reports being physically harmed. Score at least *1* if a subject reports evidence of possible physical harm. Score *2* or *3* if a rater believes that physical harm has definitely occurred based on a subject's verbal reports and behavior. Physical harm includes bruises, welts, cuts, and other physical damage, as well as being subjected to extreme physical discomfort.

136. Reports being punished a lot at home, including spanking (describe). Score at least *1* if a subject considers reported punishments to be "a lot." Score *2* or *3* depending on whether the interviewer or rater judges reported punishment as excessive.

138. Reports being sexually abused (describe). Score at least *1* if a subject reports evidence of possible sexual abuse. Score *2* or *3* if the interviewer or rater believes that sexual abuse has definitely occurred based on a subject's verbal reports and behavior. Sexual abuse can include touching and fondling of sex parts as well as more explicit sexual activity. Score item 138 for rape, but not item 217.

150. Reports concerns about family problems (describe). Score only for family problems the subject is concerned about. Examples include divorce, parental conflict, economic problems, and unsatisfactory living conditions. If a subject expresses a specific worry about a possible future event, such as divorce without indication of family problems, score item 214. Score item 215 when a subject expresses concerns about the possible death of a family member.

159. Reports disliking school or work. Score *2* or *3* only if a subject elaborates on negative feelings about school beyond an initial negative response to the interviewer's questions about school.

173. Reports getting into physical fights (except with siblings). Score for physical fights that include hitting, punching, pushing, scratching, etc. Score item 124 for verbal arguments with adults or peers without physical fighting. Score item 123 for verbal or physical fights with siblings. Score item 188 when a subject reports initiating physical attacks on other people, including siblings.

174. Reports getting teased or picked on, including by siblings. Score for physical or verbal teasing. Include reports of being called names, being ridiculed, being "put down," or being hit or punched as a form of teasing or being picked on.

176. Reports hating or disliking brother or sister. Score 2 or 3 only if a subject elaborates on negative feelings about a sibling.

184. Reports neglect of basic needs by parent or guardian (describe). Score at least *1* if a subject reports evidence of possible neglect of basic needs. Score *2* or *3* if the interviewer or rater believes that neglect has definitely occurred based on a subject's verbal reports and behavior. Basic needs include food, clothing, shelter, medical care, and education.

187. Reports obsessive thoughts (describe). Score for a subject who reports not being able to get his/her mind off a specific thought or always thinking about a specific idea. For a score of *3*, the content of the reported thoughts should be quite specific and unusual regarding an activity or object. There must be explicit preoccupation with a specific idea that intrudes into other topics. Scores of *1* and *2* can be used when there is doubt about the specificity of the preoccupation, or when the intensity or duration of the subject's report is not extreme.

188. Reports physically attacking people, including siblings. Score when a subject reports initiating a physical attack, even if the subject feels he/she was provoked. Score item 173 for reports of physical fighting without a clear attack initiated by the subject. Score item 174 for getting teased or picked on, including getting hit, when the subject does not initiate a physical attack. Do not score for hitting in the course of a physical fight, but instead score item 174.

189. Reports preferring kids older than self and *191. Reports preferring kids younger than self.* Score only for a subject's actual reports of preference for older or younger children, not just descriptions of older or younger friends.

192. Reports problems getting along with peers and *193. Reports problems making or keeping friends.* Score item 192 when a subject reports that he/she does not get along with certain children, even when he/she does get along with other children. Score item 193 when a subject reports having no friends or problems making or keeping friends. Score other more specific problems in peer relations on items 122, 134, 168, 173, or 185.

194. Reports problems with school work or job. Score for generalized complaints about school work, such as, reporting a school subject is too hard, getting poor grades, or not completing school work or homework. Score also for complaints about problems with paid jobs. Do not score for problems involving more specific learning or school problems. Score item 157 for reports of difficulty following directions. Score item 158 for difficulty learning a specific task or school subject, such as reading or math.

195. Reports running away from home. Score when a subject reports clearly having run away from home. Do not score for wishes to run away or leave home, running away from a parent in the course of discipline but then returning or getting caught, or reports that an agency removed the subject from the home (e.g., "The state took me away from home.")

198. Reports setting fires. Score *1* if limited to playing with matches or a lighter. Score *2* or *3* if a subject reports deliberately setting fires.

204. Reports teasing others, including siblings. Score *1* for playful teasing. Score *2* or *3* for more deliberate teasing or harassing, such as name calling or ridiculing others, including siblings.

207. Reports threatening other people. Score for verbal or physical threats to others. This item can include plotting revenge if a subject reports that he/she told the intended victim. Score item 218 if a subject talks about physically attacking someone, but has not actually done so or threatened the victim. Score item 220 if a subject reports seeking or planning revenge that does not include physical violence, but has not told the intended victim.

208. Reports trouble sleeping (describe). Do not score if the subject gives a plausible, specific reason or event that caused the subject to have difficulty sleeping. Examples include noises outside of the bedroom, a sibling crying, or a dog jumping on the bed or a pet needing to be let out several times a night. Score item 179 for reports of nightmares.

214. Reports worrying (describe). For scores of *2* or *3*, the content of worries must be explicitly stated, not inferred from other complaints, such as complaints about parental absence or problems with school work.

217. Reports sexual problems or excessive activity (describe). Score for sexual activity that seems unusual for age. Score item 138 for rape.

219. Talks about war or generalized violence (describe). Score descriptions of violent actions or story themes, including television shows, movies, or games if the subject's main focus is on violence. Score item 173 or item 188 for reports of actual violent actions by the subject.

228. Reports aches and pains in body. Score for aches or pains without known medical or physical cause. Score when a subject reports either past or present aches or pains occurring outside of the interview session. Do not score for aches or pains with a known physical or medical cause, such as aches or pains associated with broken bones, colds, or flu. Score item 20 for aches or pains (without known physical or medical cause) that actually occur during the interview.

229. Reports headaches. Score only for headaches without a known physical cause. Include complaints of migraines.

APPENDIX B
LOADINGS OF ITEMS ON SCICA SYNDROMES
AFTER VARIMAX ROTATIONS

Internalizing Scales
I. Anxious/Depressed^{SR}

157.	Rpts difficulty with directions	.62
160.	Rpts fearing mistakes	.59
162.	Rpts fears	.58
141.	Rpts being fearful	.57
168.	Rpts others are out to get him/her	.51
158.	Rpts difficulty learning	.49
171.	Rpts feeling worthless	.44
194.	Rpts problems with school work	.44
192.	Rpts problems getting along with peers	.44
164.	Rpts feeling guilty	.43
169.	Rpts being overtired	.43
179.	Rpts nightmares	.42
185.	Rpts not being liked	.42
137.	Rpts being self-conscious	.42
146.	Rpts being underactive	.40
134.	Rpts being lonely	.39
144.	Rpts being unable to concentrate	.38
128.	Rpts being confused	.37
214.	Rpts worrying	.34
174.	Rpts getting teased	.32
147.	Rpts being unhappy, sad, depressed	.31
193.	Rpts problems making friends	.31
	Eigenvalue	5.53

II. Anxious^{OB}

50.	Fears mistakes	.69
52.	Lacks confidence	.67
68.	Overly anxious to please	.62
83.	Self-conscious	.56
103.	Fearful	.50
65.	Nervous	.50
23.	Confused	.46
44.	Difficulty expressing self	.44
29.	Difficulty with directions	.40
102.	Concerned with neatness	.40
46.	Problems remembering facts	.38
104.	Tremors	.33
	Eigenvalue	5.45

Neither Internalizing
nor Externalizing
III. Family Problems^{SR}

186.	Rpts not getting along with parents	.69
142.	Rpts being treated unfairly at home	.61
229.	Rpts headaches	.54
234.	Rpts stomachaches	.52
177.	Rpts hating parent	.47
135.	Rpts being harmed by parent	.42
151.	Rpts concerns with neatness	.39
136.	Rpts being punished	.38
196.	Rpts screaming	.36
181.	Rpts lack of attention	.31
143.	Rpts being treated unfairly at school	.30
	Eigenvalue	3.84

IV. Withdrawn[OB]

114.	Withdrawn	.84
86.	Slow to respond verbally	.84
87.	Slow to warm up	.83
5.	Apathetic	.82
56.	Limited conversation	.79
107.	Unhappy, sad, depressed	.72
82.	Unresponsive to humor	.72
111.	Quiet	.72
106.	Underactive	.71
57.	Limited fantasy	.65
72.	Refuses to talk	.60
85.	Shy	.58
80.	Overtired	.54
79.	Secretive	.54
9.	Avoids eye contact	.53
63.	Needs coaxing	.53
77.	Says "don't know" a lot	.48
89.	Stares	.48
73.	Reluctant to discuss feelings	.47
93.	Stubborn	.35
74.	Reluctant to guess	.33
	Eigenvalue	10.43

Externalizing
V. Aggressive Behavior[SR]

188.	Rpts attacking people	.78
207.	Rpts threatening people	.66
182.	Rpts lacking guilt	.65
122.	Rpts being mean to others	.63
175.	Rpts hanging around others who get in trouble	.62
130.	Rpts disobedience at home	.60
131.	Rpts disobedience at school	.59
173.	Rpts fighting	.56
178.	Rpts hating teacher	.48
205.	Rpts temper tantrums	.44
156.	Rpts destroying others' things	.43
155.	Rpts destroying own things	.39
145.	Rpts being unable to sit still	.36
132.	Rpts being impulsive	.35
140.	Rpts being suspicious	.32
	Eigenvalue	5.80

VI. Attention Problems[OB]

53.	Lapses in attention	.52
22.	Concrete thinking	.49
4.	Acts too young	.48
42.	Clumsy	.47
32.	Doesn't sit still	.45
33.	Easily distracted	.43
88.	Speech problem	.41
64.	Needs repetition	.40
45.	Difficulty understanding	.40
24.	Reverses statements	.38
38.	Fidgets	.38
67.	Out of seat	.34
31.	Doesn't concentrate	.32
66.	Twitches	.30
	Eigenvalue	4.69

VII. Strange[OB]

92.	Strange ideas	.59
30.	Disjointed conversation	.53
15.	Brags	.50
17.	Can't get mind off thoughts	.49
35.	Exaggerates	.46
55.	Leaves to go to toilet	.46
41.	Long responses	.43
71.	Plays with sex parts	.42
16.	Burps, farts	.41
100.	Talks too much	.41
26.	Day-dreams	.39
98.	Swears	.36
91.	Strange behavior	.36
51.	Jokes too much	.35
18.	Chews clothing	.33
75.	Repeats acts	.31
3.	Giggles	.31
1.	Acts overly confident	.31
	Eigenvalue	4.91

VIII. Resistant[OB]

28.	Demands met immediately	.86
61.	Misbehaves, test limits	.84
6.	Argues	.79
48.	Impatient	.77
36.	Explosive	.76
27.	Defiant	.74
49.	Impulsive	.72
115.	Careless	.69
59.	Makes odd noises	.67
40.	Off task	.67
110.	Loud	.64
76.	Resistant	.64
10.	Irresponsible behavior	.64
112.	Wants to quit	.63
78.	Screams	.59
95.	Mood changes	.51
43.	Guesses alot	.49
60.	Messy work	.47
101.	Hot temper, angry	.45
84.	Shows off, silly	.45
105.	Manipulates	.42
97.	Suspicious	.35
21.	Complains tasks too hard	.33
99.	Talks to self	.32
7.	Asks for feedback	.31
14.	Blames interviewer	.30
	Eigenvalue	12.61

APPENDIX C
MEAN SCALE SCORES FOR REFERRED AND NONREFERRED CHILDREN AGES 6-12

Scale	T Score				Raw Score				Cronbach's Alpha[a]
	Referred		Nonreferred		Referred		Nonreferred		
	Mean	SD	Mean	SD	Mean	SD	Mean	SD	
Anxious/Depressed[SR]	52.2	9.5	47.8	6.8	11.5	7.4	8.0	4.3	.83
Anxious[OB]	51.9	12.0	49.6	8.5	6.0	5.9	4.5	3.8	.84
Family Problems[SR]	52.5	11.1	46.2	8.1	4.3	4.6	1.7	2.0	.84
Withdrawn[OB]	50.9	10.0	43.9	7.4	9.2	10.3	3.4	5.4	.86
Aggressive Behavior[SR]	51.8	10.4	44.1	7.2	5.7	5.5	2.2	2.8	.83
Attention Problems[OB]	50.7	9.6	42.0	6.7	9.5	6.0	3.7	4.4	.83
Strange[OB]	51.8	10.0	47.1	9.4	5.8	6.0	3.4	4.1	.83
Resistant[OB]	52.8	9.3	41.4	5.6	10.3	8.7	2.1	3.5	.83
Internalizing	50.6	11.3	45.8	8.9	17.5	11.2	12.5	6.5	.83
Externalizing	52.2	10.4	36.8	10.2	31.2	17.9	11.3	11.1	.81
Total-Observations	50.6	9.4	34.6	8.5	47.2	19.6	19.5	12.4	.81
Total-Self-Reports	50.8	10.2	40.6	9.5	34.7	15.4	20.8	10.2	.81

Note. N = 53 each in demographically matched referred and nonreferred samples.
[a]Cronbach's alpha computed for standardized scores.

APPENDIX D
PEARSON CORRELATIONS AMONG SCICA SCORES
REFERRED SAMPLE ABOVE DIAGONAL, NONREFERRED SAMPLE BELOW DIAGONAL

	Anx/Dep	Anxious	Fam Prob	With-drawn	Aggress	Att Prob	Strange	Resist	Int	Ext	Tot OB	Tot SR
Anx/Dep		.42	.24	-.14	.09	-.19	-.03	-.12	.88	-.11	-.03	.72
Anxious	.29		.16	.04	.03	-.22	.05	-.29	.80	-.19	.14	.40
Family Prob	.40	.16		-.15	.21	-.25	.15	.04	.27	.05	.00	.66
Withdrawn	.13	.28	-.13		-.31	-.13	-.23	.15	-.07	-.15	.49	-.32
Aggressive	.25	.18	.18	-.05		.11	.22	.12	.08	.48	.00	.49
Attention Prob	.12	-.01	.08	.00	.26		.44	.41	-.24	.72	.50	-.15
Strange	.09	-.03	.35	-.28	.25	.57		.33	.01	.71	.52	.24
Resistant	.14	-.01	.12	-.01	.45	.47	.39		-.23	.77	.71	.05
Internalizing	.83	.77	.36	.24	.26	.07	.04	.09		-.17	.05	.69
Externalizing	.19	.02	.25	-.12	.59	.82	.78	.76	.14		.69	.21
Tot OB	.25	.42	.19	.40	.34	.73	.58	.61	.41	.78		.04
Tot SR	.75	.29	.65	-.02	.62	.33	.43	.40	.67	.57	.48	

Note. Samples were demographically-matched referred and nonreferred children. N = 53 in each sample. rs ±.27 were significant at p <.05.

Library of Congress Catalogue Card #94-60044
ISBN 0–938565–32–X